THE COMPLETE NATURAL HEALING HANDBOOK

100 Step by Step Herbal Remedies to Heal Your Body Naturally
and Support Immunity Using Budget-Friendly Ingredients –
Full Color Edition (Holistic Healing Books)

Lydia Rosemont

For those beginning again:
may you find comfort in the simplest remedies,
and hear the quiet wisdom of leaves
and warm water.

Contents

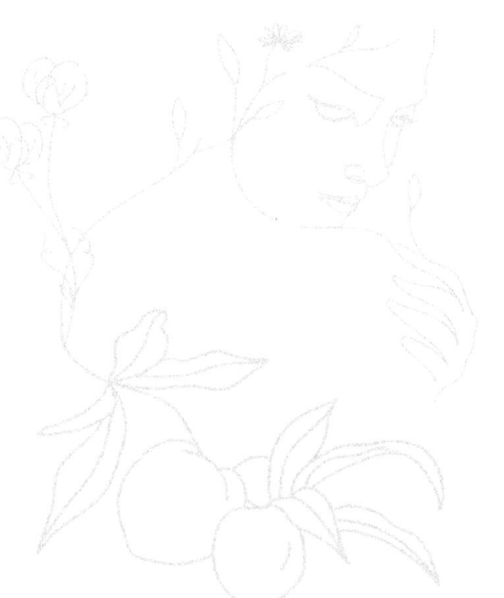

Introduction

The plants have enough spirit to transform our limited vision."

— *Rosemary Gladstar*

I want to begin by asking you a question. Have you ever stood in your kitchen late at night, staring at a half-empty box of herbal tea, and wondered if it could really make a difference? Perhaps you have read online that chamomile tea or valerian tincture can help with sleep or that peppermint and fennel soothes digestion, but you are not quite sure how to prepare it, how much to use, or whether it will actually work. Maybe you have gone down the rabbit hole of wellness blogs and social media accounts, only to leave feeling more confused, and likely more overwhelmed, than when you started. One article promises quick fixes while another warns of danger.

I know this feeling well because I once lived it myself. In my late thirties, I was exhausted nearly all the time. My body seemed to be caught in a revolving door of colds, flus, and digestive discomfort. I pushed through the days with coffee or a matcha in hand, trying to keep up with my career, my family, and the demands of modern life and our frayed and frankly disconnected society. Every single evening, I collapsed into bed wondering why my health felt so fragile. Doctors offered prescriptions and supplements that dulled my symptoms for a while, but the underlying

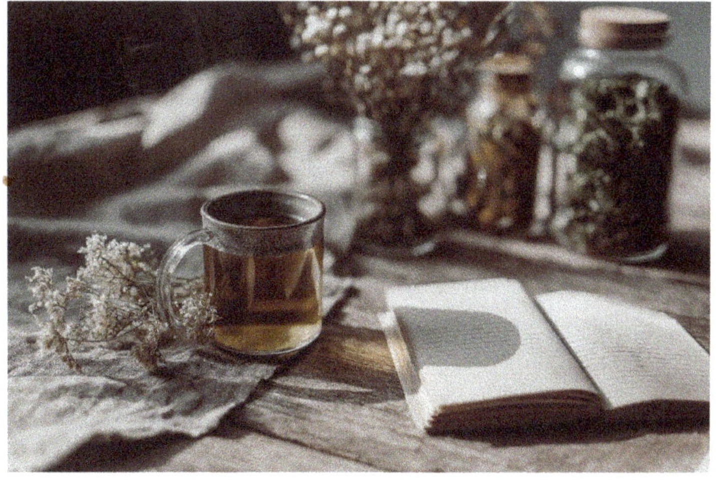

imbalance remained and my emotional health took a turn for the worse. Deep down, I longed for a more lasting solution where my body was a garden that was blooming, not a machine with many band aids.

One winter evening, as I looked over yet another bottle of over-the-counter medicine, I felt a quiet but insistent voice rise up inside me: There has to be another way!

That voice carried me back to the roots of my childhood in Vermont. I grew up surrounded by green rolling hills, maple trees, and the quiet rhythms of the countryside.

My grandmother was the first person who showed me that plants are more than just background scenery. To her, they were her closest friends and allies. She knew which leaves and flowers to pick for a fever, which roots to simmer for strength, which plant could calm a restless mind. I remember summer afternoons when she would lead me into her garden, her hands weathered from decades of tending soil, and show me how to gather chamomile blossoms one by one. She would dry them carefully in a woven basket, explaining how each plant carried its own story and purpose. At the time, I simply thought it was "Grandma's way." As an adult, I realized it was timeless wisdom that held the power to transform my health.

When I began turning back toward these remedies, I noticed small but significant changes. A cup of lemon balm and tulsi holy basil tea in the evening allowed me to ease my anxiety and rest more deeply than I had in years. A spoonful of elderberry and rosehip syrup helped me ward off the seasonal colds that always seemed to linger. My digestion improved with simple bitters made from herbs I could grow on my windowsill! This amazed me. These were not quick fixes that masked my symptoms. They were instead gentle yet powerful tools that supported my body's own capacity (and right!) to heal.

As I restored my health, I began sharing what I was learning with my family. My children, who are now grown, still remember the jars lined up on our kitchen shelves: salves for scrapes, teas for upset stomachs, syrups for coughs. My husband, who once teased me about "witchy brews," now asks me for a cup of tea whenever he feels under the weather. My mother, who still tends her own herb garden in Vermont, delights in knowing that the wisdom she passed to me through my grandmother continues to live on. That is how it is meant to be.

Eventually, what began as a personal journey became my calling. I had already worked for years as a nutritionist, but I felt drawn to teach more about natural remedies in a way that everyday people could understand. I started leading small workshops in my coastal town in Oregon, where I now live surrounded by forests and the vibrant hum of our farmers' market community.

I remember one autumn afternoon when a group of young mothers gathered in the community center. We set out bowls of dried elderberries, rosehips, ceylon cinnamon sticks, star anise, cloves, and jars of local honey from right down the road. I guided them through making their first batch of elderberry syrup. At the end of the workshop, one woman looked at her jar with tears in her eyes and said, "I feel like I can actually take care of my family now, I feel so empowered." That moment stays with me because it captures exactly why I decided to write this book.

So many people today want to live more naturally, but the information available often leaves them feeling defeated before they even start. Books and articles often tell you that lavender can help with sleep or peppermint with digestion but fail to explain how to prepare the remedy, what dosage is safe, or whether there are precautions to keep in mind. For example, peppermint isn't great for acid reflux, so it is really not ideal for all kinds of digestive discomforts. This kind of vague advice creates hesitation. Without clear guidance, you second-guess yourself and wonder, what if I get it wrong and hurt myself or my loved ones in the process? The result is that the remedy never even gets tried. I want to remove that uncertainty for you.

I have also seen how many books assume you have endless time, an expansive garden, or access to rare herbs. This excludes the busy professional who comes home late from work, lives in an urban environment, and just needs something simple and easy. To take this a step further; what about the parent who only has ten minutes before bedtime to prepare a remedy? What about the city dweller whose "garden" is a single pot on the windowsill? I want this book to meet you wherever you are, whether you are standing in a bustling grocery store in New York City or walking through a quiet farmer's market in Oregon and living on a ten acre homestead. Natural healing should be accessible to everyone, not only those with land, leisure, or advanced knowledge.

Another common struggle is simply knowing where to begin. Many natural healing books overwhelm readers by offering hundreds of remedies without any sense of direction. Imagine being new to herbs and opening a book to find five hundred recipes with no explanation of which ones are right for your current needs. It can feel like being dropped into a dense forest without a trail. I want this book to serve as your clear path with clear directions. We will walk through a simple roadmap together: pausing to listen to your body, nourishing yourself with remedies that are gentle and supportive, and then rebuilding your strength with practices that become part of your daily life. You will never be left wondering what step comes next.

Finally, and perhaps most importantly, I believe that healing is not just about information. It is also about connection. Too many books on natural remedies read like dry textbooks. They give you facts but no sense of relationship. Healing is personal. It is rooted in trust, in story, in remembering that you are not alone. Which is why I will share not only instructions but also stories—stories of my grandmother in Vermont, of families I have worked with in Oregon, of my own struggles and triumphs. I hope these stories remind you that you are stepping (and literally steeping!) into a tradition that is both ancient and alive, carried forward by people who care deeply about health, family, and community. We will touch upon folk and Indigenous traditions, Ayurveda, Traditional Chinese Medicine, and more.

I want you to imagine something with me. Imagine that a month from now you brew a cup of chamomile, passionflower, and lemon balm tea before bed, and for the first time in weeks, you fall into deep, restful sleep. Imagine preparing a simple jar of elderberry and licorice root syrup in your kitchen, knowing you have strengthened your family's immunity for the winter ahead. Imagine reaching for a peppermint oil rub the next time you feel a headache, and watching the tension melt within minutes. These moments are not far-off dreams. They are practical realities waiting for you to claim.

I am not a doctor in a white coat, and I do not pretend to be. What I offer you is something different. I bring more than fifteen years of study in herbalism, aromatherapy, and integrative health. I bring the years I spent working as a nutritionist, listening to clients share their struggles. I bring the afternoons teaching local families how to make remedies that empowered them to feel capable and confident. And my favorite of all, I bring my own lived experience of exhaustion, illness, trial, and healing.

Many of my fellow herbalists were led to this path by their own personal struggles with their health: If this is you, you are not alone. This book is the guide I wish I had when I sat at my kitchen table years ago, overwhelmed and searching for a better way.

Finally, healing is definitely not about perfection. It is not about doing everything right or memorizing every herb. It is about building a relationship with your body and the natural world. It is about remembering that the plants growing around us are not strangers but companions. It is about realizing that wellness does not have to be expensive, complicated, or reserved for experts.

As you read, I invite you to begin gently. Choose one remedy. Form a relationship with the herbs. Speak to them like your best friend, and get to know their physical and energetic qualities. Make one cup of tea. Prepare one small jar of syrup. Notice how your body responds. Healing happens in these small, steady steps. Over time, they weave together into a stronger, more vibrant life.

Welcome to The Complete Natural Healing Handbook. May this book become a resource, a companion, and a symbol of reciprocity with the plant realm. Let us begin!

CHAPTER ONE

Your Call to Healing & Your First Tea Ritual

> As we walk this plant path and gather medicine from the heart of Nature, it begins to sprout and grow within us into a living inner forest where we ourselves become the medicine."
>
> — *Sajah Popham, School of Evolutionary Herbalism*

There is a moment in every life when the body calls out for something more. Sometimes it comes as a dull ache at the back of the skull after too many days spent staring at screens. Sometimes it is the heaviness in the chest when stress or heartbreak or grief piles higher and higher, leaving no space to breathe. For some, it comes in sleepless nights, lying awake while the mind churns with worries and insomnia. For others, it is an endless fatigue that seeps into the bones, no matter how many hours of rest they try to gather. While others have endless inflamed skin that affects confidence and self-love. These signals are not random. They are the language of the body, whispering, then nudging, then insisting: It is time to pause, to listen, to heal.

I call this moment your true call to self-healing.

I remember the night mine became too loud to ignore. I was thirty-eight years old, sitting in my kitchen in Oregon, surrounded by the quiet hum of the refrigerator and the scattered remnants of another long day. In front of me was a small orange bottle of over-the-counter medicine. I had swallowed those tablets countless times before. They dulled the headaches, eased the cramps, muted the discomforts in my digestion, but they never ever touched the root. That night, as I stared at the bottle, I felt the ever-present mixture of frustration, grief, confusion, and sorrow. Was this the best I could hope for? Symptom after symptom, pill after pill, a life strung together by temporary relief? A forever band-aid? I felt disconnected from my body, mind, and spirit.

At the same time, new feelings rose up: determination and devotion. I remembered the notebook I kept as a girl in Vermont, scribbling notes while following my grandmother into the garden. She showed me how to gather chamomile blossoms, soft and golden, and dry them on a screen in the sun. She taught me how to chew a plantain leaf and place it on a bee sting to draw out the pain. She explained that peppermint leaves could clear a sharp headache and soothe an uneasy stomach. At the time, I thought of it as her peculiar, witchy, grandmother wisdom. She reminded me of the elderly women who lived in a cabin deep in the woods in the fairytale books I read. As an adult, facing my own health struggles, I realized her wisdom was now my only lifeline.

That memory opened a door. I began to reach for herbs again, tentatively at first, unsure if I remembered enough. I brewed anise hyssop and red clover tea, not from a box but from whole leaves and blossoms I bought at the local farmers' market. I simmered hawthorn berries with cinnamon and honey, surprised at how quickly my children, now nearly grown, asked for spoonfuls to keep their hearts happy. I experimented with lemon balm, planting it in a pot on my windowsill so I could harvest fresh leaves for tea to soothe my worries and stress. With consistency and deliberate choices in herbs and mindfulness around taking care of my body in other ways, I slowly and gently began to feel better. My sleep deepened. My digestion settled. The colds that once lingered for weeks became shorter and milder. My immune system felt strong and bolstered.

Most of all, I felt an emotional shift. I was no longer waiting for someone else to fix me. I was participating in my own healing, and I could track new sensations in my body as they arose. I wasn't relying on a doctor, I was relying on the medicine of the green world and my relationship and reciprocity with the plant beings. That small act of empowerment changed everything.

Why More People Are Turning Back to Nature

My story is not unique. All over the world, people are reaching for the same remedies our grandparents once trusted. People who are weary of prescriptions that cause side effects, people who feel unseen by rushed appointments, and people who long for gentler and more affordable options are turning to herbal remedies.

I have met these people in my workshops and my community. A young mother from Portland once told me that every time her toddler had another ear infection, she felt torn. She was grateful for antibiotics when they were truly needed, but she hated that they seemed to be the only option offered. She wanted tools that she could try first. She wanted gentle remedies she could prepare with her own hands. Another participant, a man in his fifties, shared that he had relied on prescription sleep aids for years. They knocked him out but left him foggy and disconnected the next day. When he learned how to make a simple custom tea for his constitution of passionflower, lemon balm, tulsi, and licorice root, and to pair it with an evening ritual of breathing, he said it was the first time in years he had felt rested and clear.

In each of these stories, the theme is the same. People are not rejecting medicine outright, but they are reclaiming balance. They are remembering that healing can be simple. They are discovering that remedies do not have to be complicated, expensive, or reserved for experts.

You Are Not Broken – You Are Just Ready for a Reset!

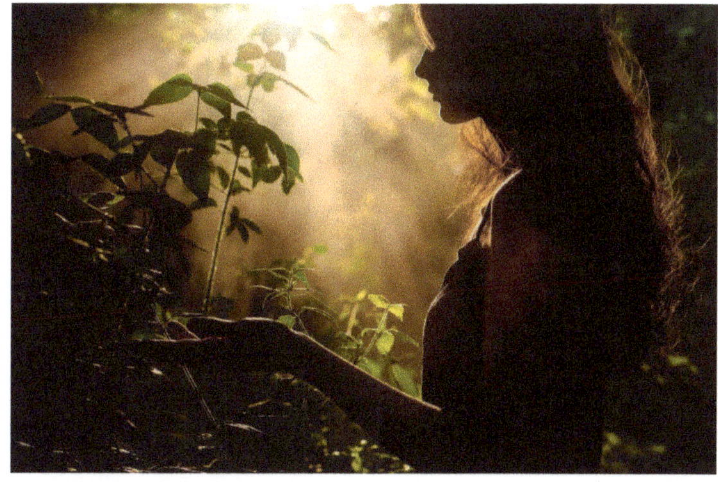

Perhaps you see yourself in these stories. Maybe you feel tired, anxious, or run-down. Maybe you have tried to piece together answers from articles and blogs, only to end up more confused. It is easy to believe that something inside you has failed. I want to say this as clearly as I can: You are not broken.

The fatigue, the headaches, the restless nights—they are not failures. They are signals. They are your body's way of saying, "Slow down. Reset. Begin again. Take Better Care of Yourself." Healing begins not with self-criticism but with compassion and slowness. It begins by listening to your body as you would to a trusted friend.

When I began to see my own symptoms this way, everything changed. Instead of pushing harder, I paused. Instead of asking, "What is wrong with me?" I began asking, "What is my body asking for?" That simple shift opened the door to real healing.

A Quick Win: The Five-Minute Grounding Tea Ritual

To help you feel this shift yourself, I want to share a ritual you can begin today. It is simple yet powerful.

Take a few teaspoons of dried chamomile, tulsi holy basil, lemon balm, and/or rose petals. Place them in a cup and pour over hot water. Let the herbs steep for five minutes. As the steam rises, close your eyes and breathe deeply. Place both feet firmly on the floor. Inhale slowly through your nose, exhale through your mouth, and imagine roots extending from your feet into the earth. Repeat three times. When the tea is ready, sip slowly. Notice the warmth as it moves through your body. Notice the way chamomile softens tension, how lemon balm lightens the mood, how tulsi helps you breathe a little easier, and how rose opens the heart. Notice how, in just a few minutes, you feel calmer, more centered, more yourself.

This is not just tea. It is an act of grounding, a declaration that you are willing to care for yourself. Chamomile contains gentle compounds that soothe the nervous system, easing anxiety and preparing the body for rest. Lemon balm has been shown in studies to calm the mind, improve mood, and support digestion. Tulsi is an adaptogen supporting stress resilience as well as the respiratory system. Rose supports antioxidants and the heart space. Together, they form a cup that nourishes body and spirit.

You do not need a vast garden or expensive tools to do this. You need only a cup, hot water, and a willingness to pause. That is the gift of herbal remedies: they meet you where you are.

From Vermont Gardens to Oregon Markets

When I sip this tea, I think of my grandmother in Vermont, bending over her garden rows, her hands stained with soil. I think of the summers when she would place fresh chamomile blossoms in my palm and say, "These will help you sleep, my girl."

I also think of my present life in Oregon, walking through the farmers' market on Saturday mornings. The air is salty from the ocean, sweet from the fresh berries, alive with chatter. Tables overflow with herbs: basil, sage, monarda, lemon balm, chamomile, thyme. I fill my basket and feel connected to something ancient and immediate all at once. These plants are not exotic. They are not far away. They are here, in our gardens, in our markets, in our kitchens.

Building Confidence, One Step at a Time

When people first begin exploring natural healing, they often hesitate. They worry they might do something wrong. They wonder if the remedies will actually work. I remind them that herbs are generous teachers. They are forgiving. Starting with something as simple as a tea ritual builds confidence. With each cup, you remember that you are capable. You learn that healing is not about mastering everything at once. It is about beginning, gently, right where you are.

Preview of the Journey Ahead

This book will guide you through a simple roadmap. You will learn to pause, to nourish, and to rebuild. You will discover remedies that soothe stress, ease digestion, strengthen immunity, and restore balance. You will see that healing is not about complexity but about connection.

Before we move into that framework, I want you to hold onto this truth: Healing is possible. It begins not in a pharmacy, not in a distant future, but in the present moment, in a cup of tea, and in the willingness to listen to your body.

Why Simple Rituals Matter

People often come to me feeling paralyzed by information. They've read articles online, tried to watch videos, even bought a few books, only to close them in frustration because the instructions felt overwhelming or the ingredients too rare. I want to remind you that healing is not about complexity. It is about presence. It is about the simple act of doing something with your own two hands, something that invites the body to exhale.

This is why the grounding tea ritual matters. It may feel small, but it begins to retrain your nervous system. When you pause long enough to steep herbs in hot water, when you breathe slowly instead of rushing to the next task, you are signaling safety to your body. That signal is powerful.

A Second Quick Win: Morning Lemon Water with Fresh Herbs

Because I know how much confidence grows with each success, I want to offer you a second quick win to begin your journey. This one is for the morning, when energy can feel sluggish and the mind is still foggy from sleep.

Fill a glass with warm water—not cold, not hot, but gently warm. Squeeze in the juice of half a lemon. If you have fresh herbs on hand, add a few sprigs of mint or a slice of fresh ginger. Stir gently. As you sip, imagine you are greeting your body with kindness. The lemon stimulates digestion and gently alkalizes the system. Mint clears the head and refreshes the breath. Ginger warms the circulation and encourages vitality. Drinking a warm drink every morning is a key in Ayurveda, the ancient holistic healing system of India and Nepal.

This ritual takes less than three minutes, yet it sets the tone for the entire day. Instead of rushing headlong into stress, you begin by choosing care. Instead of grabbing coffee first thing and pushing your nervous system into overdrive, you start with something that hydrates, awakens, and restores.

Your Body is A Garden

Why do these small shifts matter so much? I like to think of it as tending a garden. You don't restore a neglected garden overnight. You don't simply throw down seeds and expect instant blooms. You begin by loosening the soil, pulling a few weeds, watering gently, and waiting. Over time, the plants strengthen, the blossoms open, and life flourishes again. Your body is no different. Small, consistent acts of care create an environment where healing can take root.

Looking Ahead!

As you continue through this book, you will see that we will walk this path step by step. We will begin with pausing; to quiet the noise and listen to your body. We will move into nourishing; with herbs and foods that restore strength. And then we will rebuild; with practices that become part of your daily life, creating a foundation of resilience. This roadmap will keep you from feeling lost or overwhelmed. It will show you that you can begin small and grow with confidence.

But before we move forward, I want you to linger here a little longer. Take this chapter as an invitation to start now, not later. Brew the grounding tea. Try the morning lemon water. Notice the difference in your body. Feel the relief of knowing you are not broken but simply ready for a reset. Allow these practices to remind you that healing is not only possible but already unfolding the moment you choose it.

Key Takeaways

* The call to self-heal is the moment when your body's signals become too loud to ignore.
* You are not broken. Your symptoms are invitations to reset and restore. Herbal remedies are safe, effective, and accessible to everyone, not just experts.
* Healing is not dramatic—it begins with small, consistent acts like tea rituals or morning tonics.
* Science confirms what tradition has always known: Herbs like chamomile, lemon balm, ginger, and lemon gently shift the body toward balance.
* Healing is both personal and ancestral; you are reconnecting with wisdom that has always been here.

Action Steps

Today, prepare the grounding tea ritual with your herbs of choice. Drink it slowly, noticing how your body responds. Tomorrow morning, begin the day with warm lemon water infused with mint or ginger. Write a reflection after each ritual, even just a single line, about what shifted in your body or your mood. These are your first steps in answering the call to self-healing. Carry these practices with you into the next chapter, where we will explore the three-stage roadmap of Pause, Nourish, and Rebuild—the foundation of your natural healing journey.

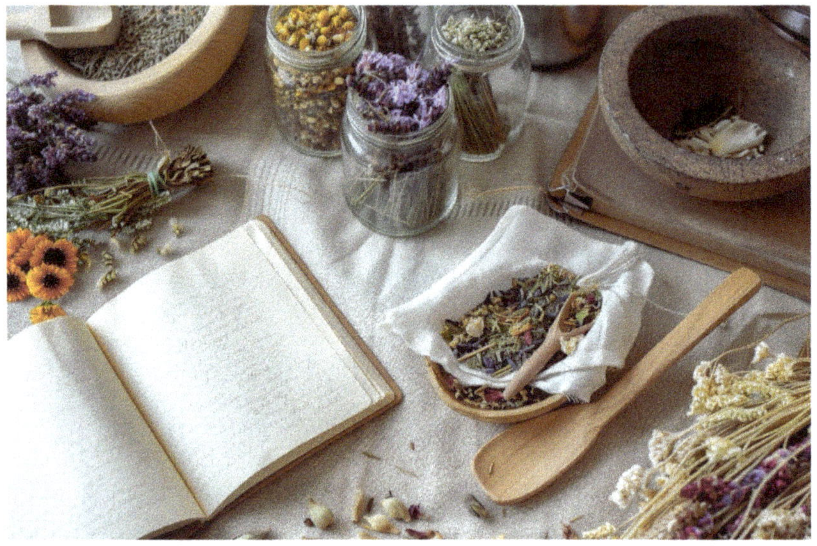

Bonus Content

You've learned the Pause, Nourish, Rebuild roadmap. Now turn it into action. Scan the QR to download the **15 Herb Starter Kit for Busy Lives**, a cheat-sheet to stock a beginner's home apothecary and get fast, practical results even on your busiest days.

CHAPTER TWO

Your Roadmap to Herbalism

> "Our sorrows and wounds are healed only when we touch them with compassion."
>
> *— Jack Kornfield*

When people first come to natural healing, their most common feeling is not excitement but overwhelm. They open a book and see hundreds of recipes. They scroll through articles that list dozens of herbs with exotic names. They look at online apothecaries and wonder if they need to buy everything at once, and some people do! Herbalism can be exciting in that way. There are so many herbs to try. However, if I were to give you one piece of advice on learning herbs—I say to pick five per year to get to know in an intimate way.

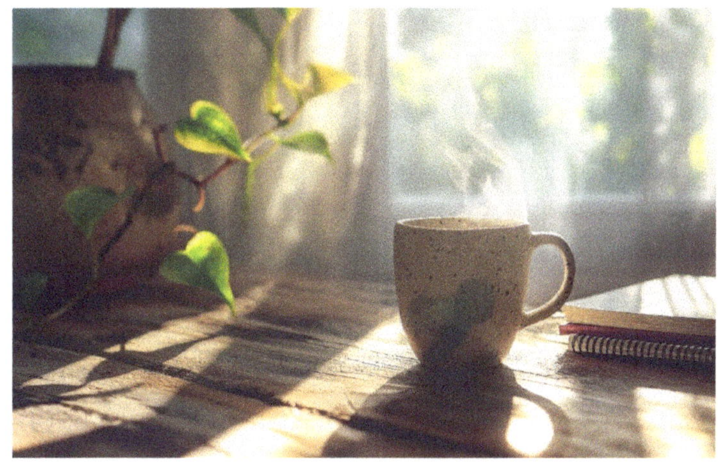

When I returned to herbal remedies in my late thirties, I filled shelves with jars, bought every herb I could find, and soon found myself exhausted and unsure of what to do next. I didn't need more herbs. I actually needed structure and simplicity. I needed a way to begin that felt possible and steady. I learned that knowing all of the intricate qualities of one herb was far more valuable than barely knowing anything about hundreds of herbs. This realization led me to create the framework that now forms the foundation of this book: Pause, Nourish, Rebuild.

Stage One: Pause

To pause is to step out of the noise and give the body space to be heard. This is harder than it sounds. Our culture rewards constant motion, endless productivity, and the belief that doing more is the solution to every problem. Unfortunately, the body does not heal when it is pushed harder. It heals when it is given permission to rest.

Herbs that support this stage are the ones that calm, ground, and restore. Passionflower for the racing mind. Skullcap for frazzled nerves. Lavender for quiet evenings. Lemon balm for anxious restlessness. These plants do not numb or sedate the way pharmaceuticals might. They invite balance. They whisper to the nervous system: You are safe, you can soften, you can let go.

I once taught a young college student who came to me overwhelmed by exams and social pressures. She told me she could barely eat from stress and her sleep was restless. I guided her to prepare a simple infusion of skullcap each evening while turning off her phone for an hour before bed. Within a week, she reported that she felt calmer, her appetite returned, and she finally slept through the night. The transformation wasn't magic, it was actually the power of pausing with the help of a gentle herb.

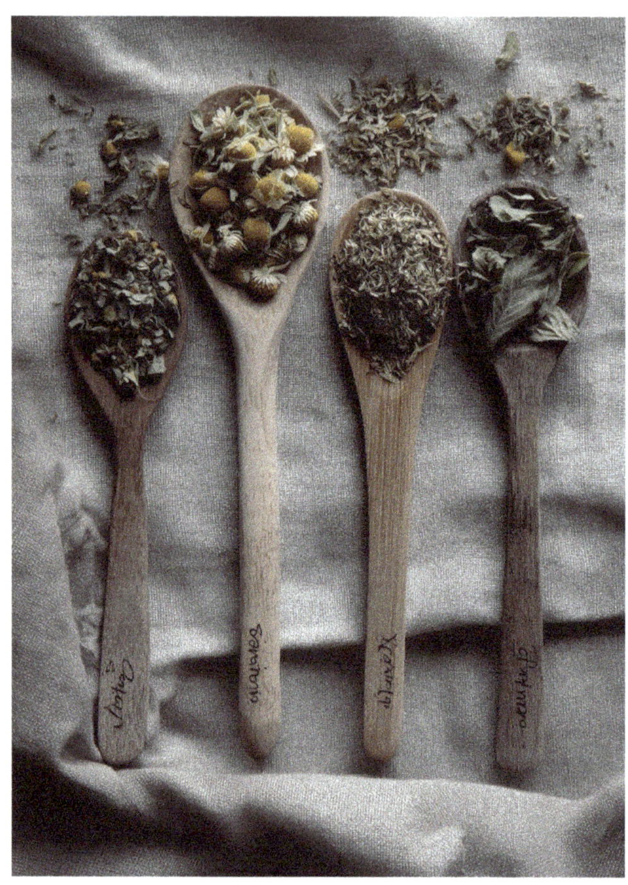

Recipe: Evening Lavender & Skullcap Tea

Steep one teaspoon dried lavender blossoms and one teaspoon dried skullcap in a cup of hot water for ten minutes. Strain and sip slowly. The floral aroma of lavender soothes the senses while skullcap eases nervous tension. This tea is especially supportive for people who hold stress in their shoulders and jaw.

Stage Two: Nourish

Once you have created space through pausing, the body asks to be nourished. Stress and illness are depleting. They draw down reserves of minerals, weaken immunity, and leave us running on empty. Nourishing herbs act like food. They restore what has been lost and rebuild the inner well.

My daily ally in this stage is nettles. Nettles are extremely rich in calcium, magnesium, iron, and protein, nettles strengthen bones, hair, skin, and energy. Another favorite is oatstraw, which gently supports the nervous system while delivering minerals. Red clover brings nourishment while also supporting hormone balance. These herbs are not quick fixes. Their magic comes from steady and long-term use. I love a long, overnight infusion of these herbs. It is a dark, dark green by morning—so mineral rich and nourishing!

Recipe: Nourishing Infusion

Place one ounce of dried nettle leaf in a quart jar. Cover with boiling water, cap, and steep for four hours or overnight. Strain in the morning. Drink throughout the day. The deep green flavor may take getting used to, but over time, many people report clearer skin, more stable moods, and a profound sense of grounded vitality.

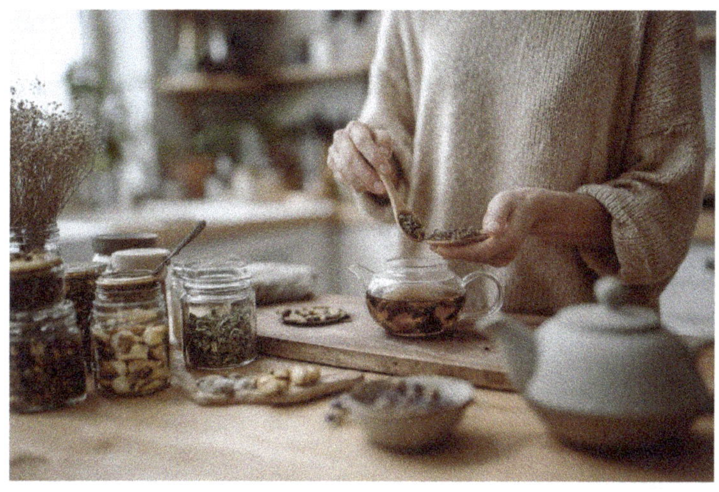

I once worked with a mother of three who was utterly depleted. Coffee had become her lifeline, yet it left her jittery and anxious. I encouraged her to try nettle infusions daily for a month and to swap her coffee for a gentler alternative like matcha. At first she doubted such a simple tea could help, but when she returned to see me four weeks later, she said, "I don't crash in the afternoon anymore. I still drink my morning coffee, but I don't need three cups just to function."

That is the power of nourishing herbs!

Stage Three: Rebuild

Finally, we move into rebuilding. This is the stage where small habits crystallize into lifestyle. Where we begin to strengthen systems of the body for the long run. Herbs here include adaptogens like ashwagandha, eleuthero, schisandra berries, shatavari, and tulsi holy basil, as well as immune allies like echinacea, thyme, rosehips, astragalus, reishi mushroom, and elderberry.

Rebuilding isn't about crisis care. It's about laying a foundation. One of my own daily rituals is stirring a teaspoon of ashwagandha root powder into warm milk with honey at night. Over time, this tonic has given me deeper sleep and stronger energy reserves during stressful seasons.

Recipe: Ashwagandha Milk

Simmer one cup of milk (dairy or plant-based) with one teaspoon of ashwagandha root powder for five minutes. Sweeten with honey and drink before bed. Ashwagandha calms the nervous system, restores the adrenals, and supports resilience.

Another simple remedy in this stage is elderberry syrup for immunity. Elderberries are rich in antioxidants and flavonoids that strengthen the body's defenses. Taking a spoonful daily during the cold months helps prevent infections or shortens their duration.

Recipe: Elderberry Syrup

Simmer one cup of dried elderberries with four cups of water, a ceylon cinnamon stick for blood sugar regulation and warming spice, a sprinkle of rosehips for vitamin C, and a few slices of fresh ginger for forty-five minutes. Strain, then stir in one cup of raw honey once cooled. Store in the refrigerator for up to two months.

Preventing Paralysis with a Starter Checklist

Beginners often ask me, "Which herbs should I buy first?" My answer is always the same: start small. A handful of versatile herbs is all you need to cover the basics. Lemon balm, lavender, nettles, oatstraw, peppermint, elderberries, echinacea, and thyme form a perfect beginner's apothecary. With these, you can make teas for stress, infusions for nourishment, syrups for immunity, and steams for colds.

You do not need special tools. A mason jar, a pot for boiling water, and a strainer are enough. Herbal healing isn't about perfection. It's about practice.

A Quick-Start Remedies Chart

- Stress → Lemon balm, skullcap, lavender, tulsi holy basil
- Fatigue/Resilience → Nettles, oatstraw, ashwagandha, tulsi holy basil, eleuthero, red clover, shatavari
- Sleep → Passionflower, valerian, lavender, skullcap, chamomile
- Immunity → elderberry, echinacea, thyme, rosehips, reishi, astragalus

Tracking Your Progress

Healing unfolds over time. To keep yourself motivated, I suggest choosing three simple actions each week. Brew a tea every evening for stress and sleep support relief. Prepare one quart of nourishing infusion to drink in the morning and throughout the day. Make a batch of elderberry syrup and take it daily. Write down how you feel at the end of the week. Small actions accumulate. They build momentum. They prevent paralysis and create confidence.

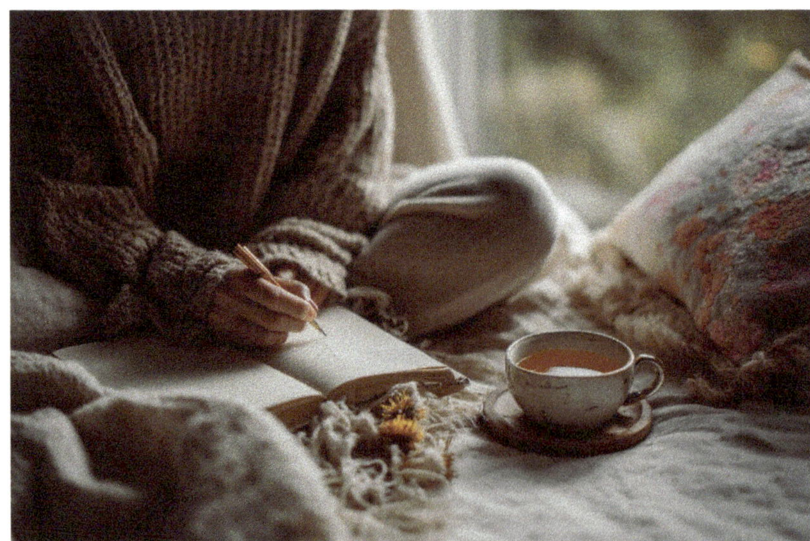

Key Takeaways

- Healing unfolds in three stages: Pause, Nourish, Rebuild.
- Pausing helps calm the nervous system with herbs like passionflower, skullcap, and lavender.
- Nourishing replenishes minerals and vitality with herbs like nettle, oatstraw, and red clover.
- Rebuilding creates long-term resilience with adaptogens like ashwagandha and immune herbs like elderberry and echinacea.
- You only need a few simple tools and a handful of herbs to begin.
- Consistency, not complexity, is the key to progress.

Action Steps

This week, choose three practices. Brew an evening tea of lavender and skullcap to pause. Prepare a quart of nettle infusion at the same time so you are prepared for the next day. Make a batch of elderberry syrup to rebuild. Write down how you feel after each practice. Notice what shifts in your body and your mood, how the herbal scents waft through your kitchen. Carry this sense of empowerment into the next chapter, where we will dive deeper into the art of creating your own home apothecary.

CHAPTER THREE

Building Your First Home Apothecary

"Herbal medicine-making is much like dancing; it's easy, it's natural, and it's undeniably delightful. To say the least, it is a lucid expression of one's distinct character."

— *Herbalist James Green*

I still remember the first time I opened a cupboard in my grandmother's Vermont kitchen and found what she called her "apothecary." It wasn't fancy. No carved shelves or ancient jars. Just simple glass containers lined up in a row, each with a hand-written label. Chamomile, sage, calendula, yarrow, peppermint… a pot of oil infusing with rosemary sat by the sunny window, and a mortar and pestle rested on the counter. From this small collection, she created endless remedies: teas for colds, gargles for sore throats, salves for cuts and scrapes.

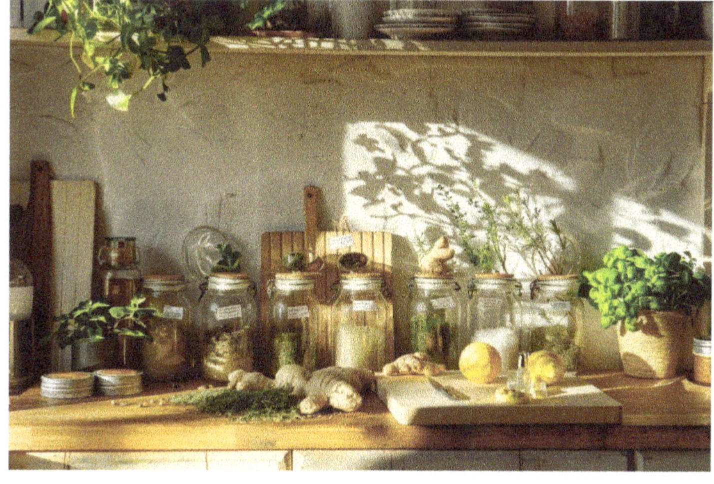

That memory taught me something I've never forgotten: You don't need a massive collection of herbs to begin. You need a **starter kit**! A handful of reliable plants that cover your everyday needs, some jars to store them, and the knowledge of how to use them. Over time, you'll add more, but the foundation is simple.

This chapter is your guide to building that foundation, your true home apothecary.

Fifteen Must-Have Herbs for Your Starter Kit

Here are fifteen versatile herbs to begin with. Together, they cover stress, sleep, digestion, immunity, inflammation, wounds, emotional balance, and general vitality.

1. Calendula (Calendula officinalis)

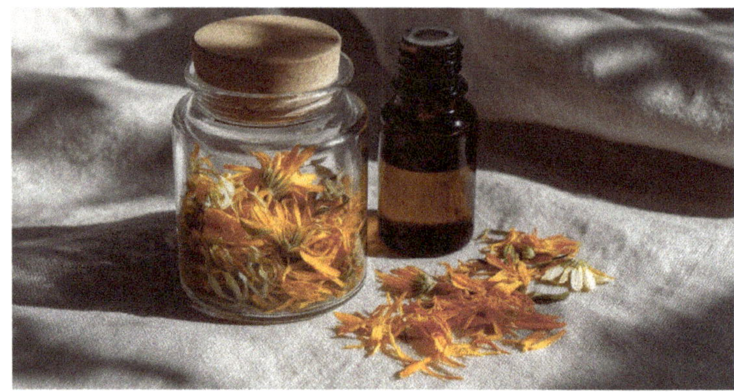

I think of calendula as sunshine in a bottle. It has golden-orange petals that brighten the garden and bring lightness to the spirit. My grandmother used it often for cuts and rashes but also for what she called "stuckness" in the body. Calendula gently moves the lymphatic system, helping the body clear waste and restore flow.

- **Medicinal uses:** Wound healing, rashes, dry skin, lymphatic support, digestive inflammation.
- **Best beginner form:** Dried petals for teas, oils, or salves.
- **Store-bought alternative:** Calendula salves, creams, and diaper ointments.
- **Urban hack:** Calendula grows beautifully in pots or wild in the garden. Scatter seeds on a balcony or windowsill planter or in your garden beds for blooms all summer. Dead-head and they'll produce more flowers.

Recipe: Calendula Healing Oil

Fill a clean glass jar halfway with dried calendula petals. Cover with olive oil. Cap and place in a sunny window for 3–4 weeks, shaking daily. Strain and store in a dark jar. Use for cuts, scrapes, diaper rash, or chapped skin.

2. Rosemary (Rosmarinus officinalis)

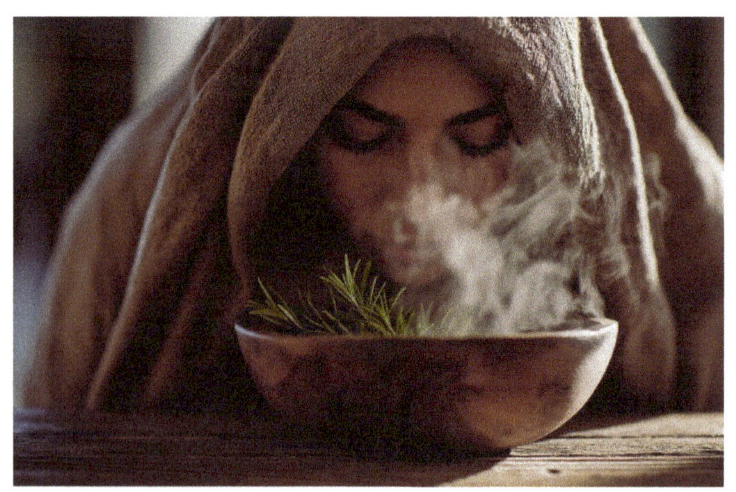

Rosemary has been called the herb of remembrance. Its scent wakes up the mind, improves focus, and stimulates circulation. In my coastal Oregon kitchen, I always keep a jar of rosemary sprigs drying. I reach for it on foggy mornings when my thoughts feel sluggish, and it immediately awakens my brain!

- **Medicinal uses:** Improves memory, circulation, relieves muscle aches, clears congestion.

- **Best beginner form:** Fresh or dried sprigs for tea and steam.
- **Store-bought alternative:** Rosemary essential oil for topical use.
- **Urban hack:** Keep a rosemary shrub in a pot, it doubles as medicine and seasoning.

Recipe: Rosemary Steam for Congestion

Place a handful of fresh rosemary in a bowl. Pour over boiling water. Drape a towel over your head and breathe the steam for 5–10 minutes. This clears sinuses and eases colds.

3. Yarrow (Achillea millefolium)

Named after Achilles, who is said to have used it on the battlefield, yarrow is a powerful wound herb. Its feathery leaves stop bleeding quickly, while its flowers support the body in releasing fevers. Its flower essence is supportive for keeping strong energetic boundaries.

- **Medicinal uses:** Wound care, fever support, circulatory health, energetic boundaries
- **Best beginner form:** Dried flowers and leaves.
- **Store-bought alternative:** Yarrow tea blends.
- **Urban hack:** Yarrow grows wild along roadsides and lawns—just be sure of correct identification before harvesting.

Recipe: Yarrow Fever Tea

Blend 1 tsp yarrow, 1 tsp peppermint, and 1 tsp elderflower. Steep 10 minutes. Drink hot to encourage sweating and reduce fever gently.

4. Garden Sage (Salvia officinalis)

Garden sage is both food and medicine. My grandmother used it for sore throats. Sage has antimicrobial and astringent properties.

- **Medicinal uses:** Sore throats, digestion, menopausal hot flashes, excess sweating.
- **Best beginner form:** Dried leaves for tea or gargles.
- **Store-bought alternative:** Sage lozenges and sprays.
- **Urban hack:** Grow sage in a small pot. Once established, it'll be with you for years.

Recipe: Sage Gargle

Steep 2 tsp dried sage in a cup of hot water for 15 minutes. Cool and gargle several times daily for sore throats.

5. Cinnamon (Cinnamomum verum)

Cinnamon adds more than flavor. It warms the body, supports circulation, and helps balance blood sugar. I use it in winter teas, often blended with ginger for immune support. Ceylon cinnamon supports blood sugar regulation.

- **Medicinal uses:** Warming spice, antimicrobial, circulatory stimulant, blood sugar support.
- **Best beginner form:** Ground or stick form from the spice aisle.
- **Store-bought alternative:** Cinnamon teas or capsules.
- **Urban hack:** Always keep a jar of cinnamon sticks. They store well and double as medicine.

Recipe: Cinnamon Ginger Honey Paste

Mix 2 tbsp ground cinnamon, 2 tbsp grated ginger, and ½ cup raw honey. Take 1 tsp daily in winter for warmth and immune support.

6. Marshmallow Root (Althaea officinalis)

Soft and soothing, marshmallow root protects and calms mucous membranes. It is invaluable for dry coughs, sore throats, and irritated digestion.

- **Medicinal uses:** Sore throats, dry coughs, heartburn, digestive irritation.
- **Best beginner form:** Dried root for cold infusions.
- **Store-bought alternative:** Herbal cough syrups with marshmallow.
- **Urban hack:** If marshmallow is unavailable, slippery elm lozenges provide similar relief.

Recipe: Marshmallow Cold Infusion

Place 2 tbsp dried root in a jar. Cover with cold water. Steep overnight. Strain and sip to soothe dryness.

7. Chamomile (Matricaria recutita)

Chamomile is gentle yet powerful. Beyond its reputation for sleep, it eases stomachaches, calms children, and relieves tension.

- **Medicinal uses:** Sleep aid, digestive support, calming nervous tension.
- **Best beginner form:** Dried flowers for tea.
- **Store-bought alternative:** Chamomile tea bags.
- **Urban hack:** Blend with lavender or lemon balm for a stronger calming effect.

Recipe: Chamomile Compress

Steep a strong cup of chamomile tea. Soak a cloth and place over irritated eyes or inflamed skin.

8. Turmeric (Curcuma longa)

Known for its golden color, turmeric is one of the best anti-inflammatory herbs. It supports joint health, liver detoxification, and digestion. It is one of Ayurveda's renowned healing medicinals.

- **Medicinal uses:** Joint pain, inflammation, liver support.
- **Best beginner form:** Fresh root or ground spice.
- **Store-bought alternative:** Golden milk powder mixes.
- **Urban hack:** Freeze fresh turmeric roots and grate as needed.

Recipe: Ayurvedic Golden Milk

Simmer 1 cup milk with 1 tsp turmeric, a pinch of black pepper, and honey. Drink before bed for inflammation and rest.

9. Rose (Rosa spp.)

Rose is medicine for the heart. Its petals calm grief, uplift the spirit, and soothe skin. I turn to rose in times of loss or stress.

- **Medicinal uses:** Emotional balance, skin healing, digestive tonic.
- **Best beginner form:** Dried petals or rose water.
- **Store-bought alternative:** Culinary rose water.
- **Urban hack:** Add petals to baths or blend into teas for emotional soothing.

Recipe: Rose Petal Tea

Steep 1 tbsp dried petals in hot water for 10 minutes. Drink for emotional grounding.

10. Garlic (Allium sativum)

Garlic may be the most humble medicine, yet it is one of the strongest and most capable. It boosts immunity, lowers cholesterol, and fights infections.

- **Medicinal uses:** Immune support, antimicrobial, cardiovascular tonic.
- **Best beginner form:** Fresh cloves.
- **Store-bought alternative:** Garlic capsules or extracts.
- **Urban hack:** Keep garlic honey ready year-round—it doubles as food and medicine.

Recipe: Garlic Honey

Peel and crush cloves. Place in a jar and cover with raw honey. Let sit 1 week. Take 1 tsp at the first sign of a cold.

11.   Nettle (Urtica dioica)

A powerhouse of minerals, nettle builds vitality and relieves allergies.

- **Medicinal uses:** Energy, bone health, allergies.
- **Best beginner form:** Dried leaf for infusion.
- **Store-bought alternative:** Nettle tea bags.
- **Urban hack:** Brew overnight in a mason jar.

Recipe: Nettle Infusion

1 oz dried nettle in a quart jar, cover with boiling water, steep overnight. Strain and drink daily.

12.   Oatstraw (Avena sativa)

Oatstraw nourishes the nervous system. I often recommend it for burnout and recovery from stress.

- **Medicinal uses:** Nervous exhaustion, nutrient replenishment.
- **Best beginner form:** Dried straw for infusions.
- **Store-bought alternative:** Calming teas with oats.
- **Urban hack:** Brew strong, chill, and sip during the workday.

Recipe: Oatstraw and Rose Infusion

Steep oatstraw overnight with a handful of dried rose petals. A tonic for emotional steadiness.

13.   Elderberry (Sambucus nigra)

One of the best herbs for immune defense.

- **Medicinal uses:** Cold and flu prevention and recovery.
- **Best beginner form:** Dried berries for syrup.
- **Store-bought alternative:** Elderberry syrups.
- **Urban hack:** Make small batches and store in the fridge.

Recipe: Elderberry Syrup

Simmer 1 cup dried berries with 4 cups water, cinnamon stick, and ginger slices. Reduce by half, strain, and add 1 cup honey. Take daily.

14.   Echinacea (Echinacea purpurea)

Stimulates immune defenses, especially at the first sign of illness.

- **Medicinal uses:** Infections, immune activation.

- **Best beginner form:** Tincture.
- **Store-bought alternative:** Capsules or tinctures.
- **Urban hack:** Keep a 1 oz dropper bottle in your bag during flu and cold season.

Recipe: Echinacea Tincture

At first sign of illness, take 30 drops every 2 hours for 24 hours, then reduce to 3x daily.

15. Tulsi / Holy Basil (Ocimum tenuiflorum)

Sacred to Ayurveda and native to the regions of India and Nepal, tulsi is an adaptogen that helps the body adapt to stress and also a beautiful respiratory ally.

- **Medicinal uses:** Stress resilience, mood uplift, immune support, respiratory support, meditative/spiritual ally.
- **Best beginner form:** Dried leaf for tea.
- **Store-bought alternative:** Tulsi tea bags.
- **Urban hack:** Grow tulsi in a pot or in garden beds. It thrives with warmth and sunlight and in climates that get more rain.

Recipe: Tulsi Iced Tea

Steep a handful of tulsi leaves in hot water. Chill and add lemon slices. A cooling summer tonic. It is my absolute favorite tea—so delicious and grounding!

Storing and Organizing Your Apothecary

When people first begin gathering herbs, one of the biggest questions I hear is: "Where do I put it all?" Many imagine they'll need a full room lined with shelves, or worry they'll never have enough space in their small kitchen apartment. The truth is, you can build an effective apothecary in a single cupboard or a makeshift space you create out of recycled materials—it is really up to you! Get creative!

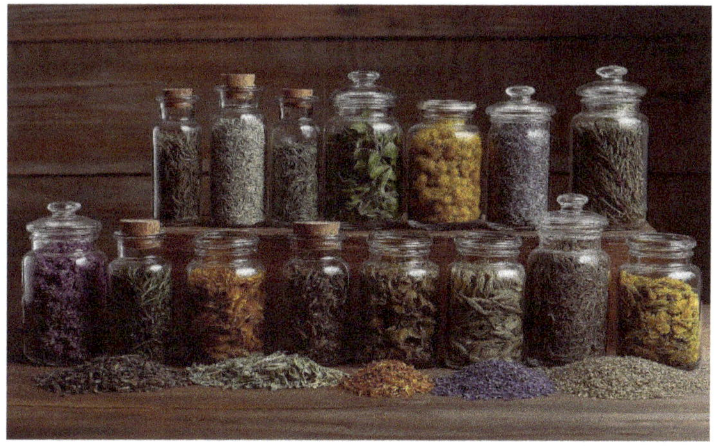

What matters most is not the size of your collection but how you care for it. Herbs are living medicine, even when dried, and they deserve to be treated with respect. A well-kept apothecary will serve you faithfully, while a neglected one that is forgotten or left out in the sunlight can leave you with stale jars and weak remedies. Let's walk through everything you need to know.

Choosing Storage Jars

Glass is the gold standard. Herbs stored in plastic quickly lose their aroma and potency, and plastic can leach chemicals over time. Clear mason jars, recycled pasta sauce jars, or wide-mouthed glass containers all work beautifully.

If your jars are clear and exposed to light, store them in a cupboard or cover them with brown paper bags to protect against fading. Light and heat are the two biggest enemies of herbal potency.

A SIMPLE RULE OF THUMB: if your herb has lost its color and scent, it has lost much of its medicine. A vibrant green nettle, a deep orange calendula petal, a sharp aromatic lemon balm leaf are signs of freshness.

LYDIA'S NOTE: On my kitchen shelf right now sits a row of recycled jam jars, each with a handwritten label. My grandmother never bought fancy jars either. She truly believed the real wealth was what was inside.

Labeling Your Herbs

It may seem obvious, but I've seen even the most experienced herbalists get caught by unlabeled jars. Once you have ten different green leaves in glass containers, you'll be surprised how similar they look.

Always label your jars with:

* *The* name of the herb *(both common and botanical, if you'd like).*
* *The* date *you purchased or harvested it.*
* *The* source *(farmers' market, garden, online apothecary).*

I like to add a note about the plant's primary use. A jar of dried lemon balm on my shelf reads: "Lemon Balm – June 2024 – Local Farm. Calm nerves and anxiety, anti-viral." It's amazing how even a few words jog memory and inspire creative use.

Shelf Life and Potency

Most dried leaves and flowers stay potent for about a year if stored properly. Roots and barks often last two to three years, since they are denser and retain compounds longer. Seeds and berries fall somewhere in between.

Signs your herbs are past their prime:

* Color is faded to brown or gray.
* Aroma is weak or nonexistent.
* Taste is dull, dusty, or flat.

Don't worry if you discover old jars. Compost them! Herbs return easily to the soil, and you can refill your jars with fresh vibrancy.

SEASONAL CHECK-IN: Twice a year (spring and autumn), I go through every jar in my cupboard. I smell, I look, I taste. Anything that feels lifeless gets offered back to the earth. This ritual keeps my apothecary alive and reminds me that medicine is always moving and never static.

Tools You Actually Need

Forget expensive equipment. A starter apothecary can run beautifully on what most kitchens already have.

- **Kettle or saucepan** – for boiling water.
- **Strainer or fine mesh sieve** – for teas and infusions.
- **Mason jars or recycled glass jars** – for storing herbs and brewing infusions.
- **Measuring spoons** – helpful for consistent results.

Optional (but lovely as you grow):

- **Mortar and pestle** – for crushing seeds or grinding roots.
- **Cheesecloth or muslin bags** – for straining oils and syrups.
- **Funnels** – to pour liquids neatly into bottles.
- **Dropper bottles** – for tinctures or glycerites.

URBAN HACK: A French press works wonderfully for brewing strong herbal teas and infusions. I've had students in tiny apartments use their coffee press exclusively for herbs.

Sourcing Herbs

Where you get your herbs matters. Look for sources that emphasize quality, freshness, and sustainability.

- **Farmers' Markets:** Fresh bundles of rosemary, sage, mint, and calendula are often available in season. This also builds relationships with amazing local growers that you can learn a lot from.
- **Online Apothecaries:** Mountain Rose Herbs, Starwest Botanicals, Frontier Co-op, and other trusted companies ship organic dried herbs in bulk.
- **Grocery Stores:** Don't overlook your spice aisle! Cinnamon sticks, ginger, turmeric, and thyme are everyday herbs with powerful medicinal use.
- **International Markets:** Middle Eastern and South Asian grocers often carry rose water, dried hibiscus, and unique spices.

LYDIA'S NOTE: I keep a blend of sources. The farmers' market for fresh bundles, my garden for mint and tulsi, and a small box of online-ordered roots tucked in the pantry. You don't need it all from one place, variety is the spice of life!

Building an Apothecary in Small Spaces

You don't need a farmhouse kitchen to create an herbal space. I've seen beautiful apothecaries in studio apartments, dorm rooms, and tiny city flats.

STORY: One of my students in Portland lived in a one-bedroom apartment with no storage space. She kept her herbs in a shoebox under the bed, neatly labeled in pint-sized jars. She told me, "Even though I only had eight jars, when I pulled that box out, it felt like opening a treasure chest."

Here are some ideas for tiny-space apothecaries:

- **Shoebox Apothecary:** Store 6–10 jars in a shoebox under the bed or in a closet.
- **Windowsill Garden:** Grow a pot of rosemary, mint, or tulsi where sunlight pours in. These herbs thrive in small pots and provide constant medicine.
- **Pantry Apothecary:** Dedicate one shelf to spices and herbs. Cinnamon, garlic, ginger, and thyme already live in most kitchens—see them as medicine too.
- **Wall Shelves:** A single shelf with 6–12 jars can transform into a miniature apothecary.

Keeping Your Apothecary Alive

An apothecary is not meant to be a museum shelf. It's meant to be alive—opened, used, replenished. Here are my favorite practices for keeping the energy flowing:

- **Rotate seasonally:** Use up herbs within a year. In spring, focus on fresh nettle, dandelion, and chickweed. In summer, rose and mint. In autumn, elderberry and echinacea. In winter, cinnamon, garlic, and turmeric.
- **Keep notes:** A simple journal where you jot what remedies you made and how they worked for you builds confidence and experience.
- **Invite beauty:** Place flowers, a candle, or a stone by your apothecary shelf. When your space feels special, you're more likely to use it.

ANECDOTE: My grandmother's shelf always had a small vase of fresh flowers next to the jars. "The plants like to be near other living things," she'd say. That little touch made her kitchen shelf feel like an altar and a sacred space, not just storage.

The Heart of a Home Apothecary

At its core, a home apothecary is not about having dozens of jars. It's about cultivating relationship. With every label you write, every jar you shake, every tea you brew, you're participating in a lineage of care.

I often tell my students: Your apothecary should feel like a friend you want to visit, not a chore you have to maintain.

Whether it's one jar of nettles or twenty jars in neat rows, your collection is a mirror of your healing journey. Let it grow slowly, season by season. Let it be humble. Let it be alive.

Key Takeaways

- Fifteen herbs are enough to build a complete and versatile starter kit.
- Each herb has multiple uses, recipes, and store-bought alternatives.
- Storage and labeling are as important as the herbs themselves.
- With just jars, a kettle, and a strainer, you can make almost any beginner remedy.
- You don't need a garden—balconies, windowsills, and even spice racks can form your apothecary.

Action Steps

Choose five herbs from this chapter and prepare one remedy from each in the next week. Journal your experiences—taste, scent, effect on your body. Begin to notice which herbs resonate with you most. These will become your closest allies. In the next chapter, we will take these herbs and expand into the art of preparing a wider range of remedies: teas, tinctures, syrups, salves, and more.

BONUS: Seasonal Rotations: Keeping Your Apothecary Alive Through the Year

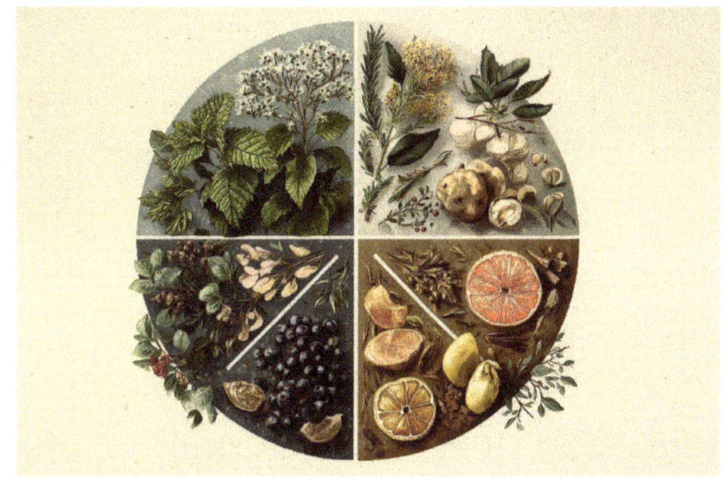

One of the most beautiful lessons the plants teach us is that healing is never static. Just as the seasons shift, so too do our bodies' needs. A summer apothecary will look different from a winter one. Herbs come into their fullest expression at different times of the year, and learning to work with this rhythm is part of what makes herbalism so alive.

When I was growing up in Vermont, my grandmother always reminded me that the jars in her cupboard were not meant to stay sealed and untouched. "They are living medicine," she would say. "Use them, share them, and when the season turns, we will gather more." That rhythm of replenishing the apothecary with the changing year is what keeps it vibrant.

Here's how to rotate and refresh your apothecary season by season.

Spring: Renewal and Clearing

Spring is the season of waking up. Our bodies often feel heavy from winter: sluggish digestion, low energy, or perhaps a lingering cough. This is the time for herbs that stimulate circulation, clear stagnation, and bring freshness.

- **Dandelion root and leaf:** Supports liver detoxification and gently stimulates digestion.
- **Nettle (fresh spring leaves):** At its most vibrant in spring, nettle floods the body with minerals and helps ease seasonal allergies.
- **Chickweed:** Cooling and moistening, perfect for skin and lymphatic support.

SPRING RITUAL: A fresh nettle soup or tea brewed from just-harvested leaves is the perfect way to align your body with spring energy.

Summer: Vitality and Cooling

Summer is abundant, and with abundance often comes heat, inflammation, and a need to stay cool and hydrated. Herbs in summer are often refreshing, aromatic, and protective against sun and stress.

- **Peppermint:** Cooling for digestion and heat-related headaches.
- **Tulsi (holy basil):** Stress resilience in the heat of busy summer days.
- **Rose petals:** Emotional soother and cooling tea for overheated bodies and hearts.
- **Calendula:** Blooms all summer, supports skin against sun exposure and minor burns.

SUMMER RITUAL: Brew a pitcher of iced rose and peppermint tea. Keep in the fridge for hot afternoons—it's refreshing, uplifting, and hydrating.

Autumn: Strengthening and Preparing

Autumn is the season of transition. Days shorten, air grows cooler, and immune challenges return. This is the time to fortify the body, support immunity, and begin slowing down.

- **Elderberry:** Syrups prepared in autumn carry you through cold season.
- **Echinacea:** Tinctures help prime immune defenses for winter.
- **Sage:** Perfect for autumn sore throats and colds.
- **Thyme:** Supports the lungs during seasonal shifts.

AUTUMN RITUAL: Simmer a pot of elderberry syrup with cinnamon and ginger. Bottle it and keep it at the front of your apothecary shelf for daily use.

Winter: Rest and Deep Nourishment

Winter is a season of rest. The body needs warmth, resilience, and steady support. Herbs in winter are often warming, immune-boosting, and deeply nourishing.

- **Cinnamon and ginger:** Keep circulation warm and digestion strong.
- **Turmeric:** Reduces inflammation and supports joints in cold weather.
- **Oatstraw and nettle:** Nourishing infusions provide minerals when fresh greens are scarce.
- **Garlic:** A winter powerhouse for immunity.

WINTER RITUAL: Prepare golden milk with turmeric, ginger, cinnamon, and honey in the evenings. It warms the body and calms the nervous system, making long nights more restful.

Refreshing Your Apothecary Seasonally

As seasons shift, check your jars. Which herbs are low? Which are stale? Which are abundant right now? Let your apothecary breathe with the seasons—use what you have, then refill with what is freshest.

In my own home, I keep a tradition of spring cleaning my jars every March. Anything faded or lifeless goes into the compost. Anything vibrant stays. In summer, I dry bundles of herbs from my garden or the farmers' market to carry into fall. In autumn, I simmer syrups and tinctures to store for winter. In winter, I lean into the jars of roots and warming spices that will carry me through.

When you build this rhythm, your apothecary becomes more than jars on a shelf. It becomes a living cycle, a reflection of nature's turning wheel, and an extension of your own body's needs.

CHAPTER FOUR

Herbal Remedies for Real-Life Relief

> "When one tugs at a single thing in nature, he finds it attached to the rest of the world."
>
> — *John Muir*

We all long for relief. Relief from the stress that weighs on our shoulders. Relief from the fog of fatigue that clouds our mornings. Relief from the restless nights when sleep feels far away. Relief from the first scratch in the throat that warns of a coming cold.

Herbs have always been there for these moments. They are the quiet companions that sit patiently on our shelves, waiting for us to remember them. Unlike a pill bottle, they invite us into ritual. Each remedy is

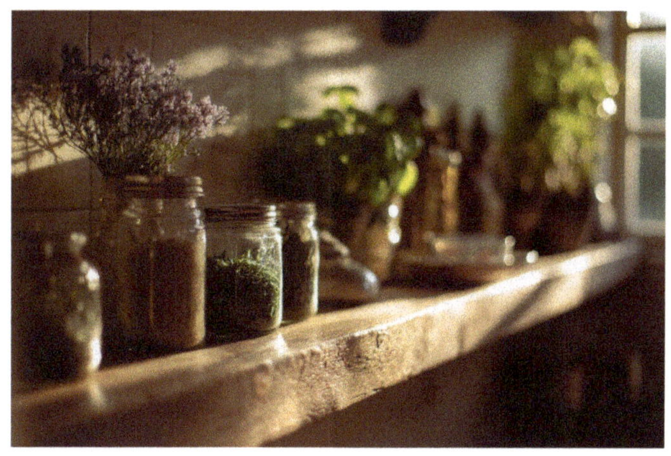

more than a recipe…it is a conversation, a slowing down, a way to place our hands back on the pulse of life.

This chapter is where your apothecary comes alive. You'll learn not just *what* herbs can do but *how* to work with them in a practical, approachable way. For each of the most common struggles, such as stress, fatigue, sleep, and immunity, I will guide you through three types of remedies:

- Daily Rituals you can weave gently into your routine, like a cup of tea or a nightly soak.

- Quick Remedies for those sudden moments when you need relief in minutes.

- Deep-Repair Remedies that rebuild resilience over weeks and months.

By the end of this chapter, you'll hold forty remedies in your hands: a full toolkit for daily life. You'll find both comfort and confidence here, knowing that with every sip, every drop, every breath of steam, you are taking part in your own healing.

Stress & Anxiety Remedies (1–10)

1. Tulsi & Lemon Balm Morning Tea

Why It Helps

Tulsi (holy basil) is an adaptogen that regulates cortisol and promotes calm focus, while lemon balm soothes anxious tension.

How to Use

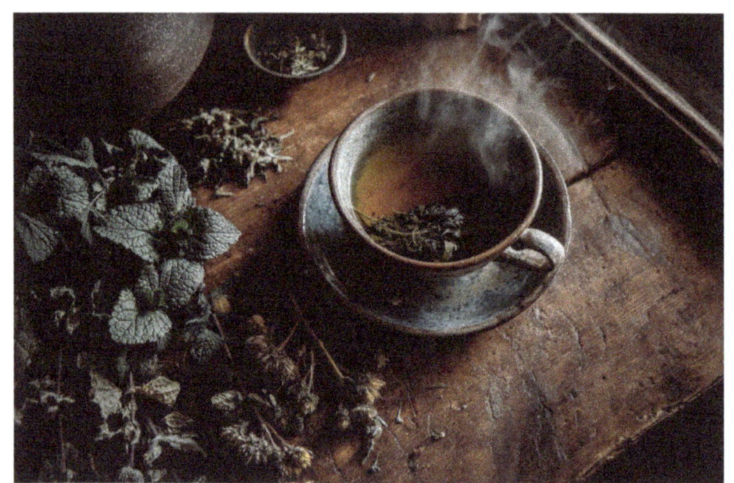

- 1 tsp dried tulsi
- 1 tsp dried lemon balm
- 2 cups hot water

  Steep 10–15 minutes, covered. Drink mid-morning or afternoon.

Quick Remedy	Safety Notes	Variations
Chill and serve over ice with lemon slices in summer.	Avoid lemon balm if you have hypothyroidism, without medical guidance.	Add peppermint for extra clarity or rose petals for emotional uplift.

2. Lavender Hand Inhalation

Why It Helps

Lavender's volatile oils act quickly on the nervous system. Research shows lavender inhalation can lower cortisol and heart rate.

How to Use

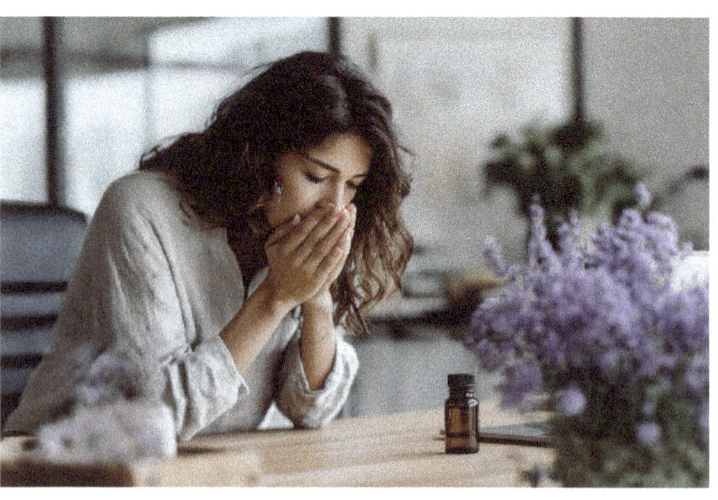

- Place 2 drops lavender essential oil on your palms.
- Rub together and cup hands over your face.
- Inhale slowly for 3 breaths.

Quick Remedy	Safety Notes	Variations
Takes less than 30 seconds— ideal for travel or work.	Avoid eye contact. Essential oils should be diluted if used on sensitive skin.	No oil? Crush rosemary or mint leaves between fingers and inhale.

3. Milky Oat Tincture

Why It Helps

Milky oats are a restorative nervine, excellent for long-term stress recovery. They nourish the nervous system rather than merely sedating it.

How to Use

* Take 30–60 drops tincture in water 2–3 times daily.
* Use consistently for several months.

Quick Remedy	Safety Notes	Variations
None—this is a deep repair remedy.	Safe for most people, but avoid if allergic to oats.	Blend with rose glycerite for grief support or skullcap tincture for irritability.

4. Rose & Oatstraw Infusion

Why It Helps

Oatstraw replenishes minerals, while rose uplifts mood and softens emotional tension.

How to Use

* 1 oz dried oatstraw
* 2 tbsp dried rose petals
* 1 quart boiling water
  Steep 4–8 hours or overnight. Strain and sip through the day.

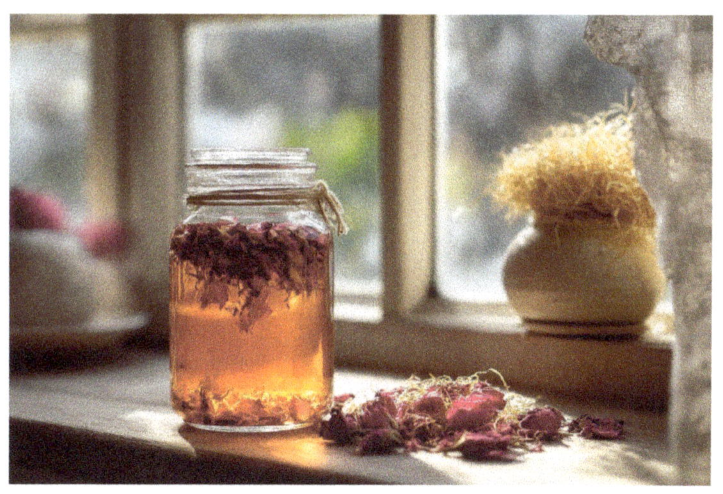

Quick Remedy	Safety Notes	Variations
Steep 1 tsp of each in a cup of hot water for 10 minutes if short on time.	Avoid roses treated with pesticides; always source organic petals.	Add chamomile for digestive calm.

5. Lemon Balm Tincture Drops

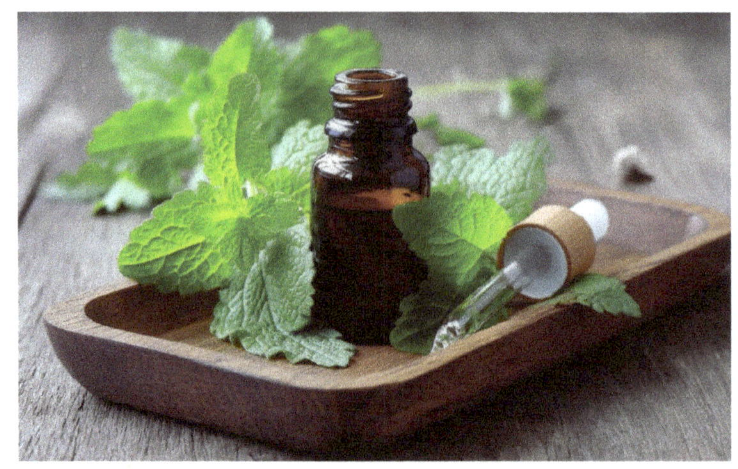

Why It Helps

Lemon balm is fast acting for anxiety, restlessness, or jitters. It also supports digestion.

How to Use

Take 30–40 drops tincture in a splash of water. Relief comes in 15–20 minutes.

Quick Remedy	Safety Notes	Variations
Keep a 1-oz bottle in your bag for commutes or crowded spaces.	Not recommended in large doses for those with hypothyroidism.	Combine with skullcap for more grounding effect.

6. Ashwagandha Honey Paste

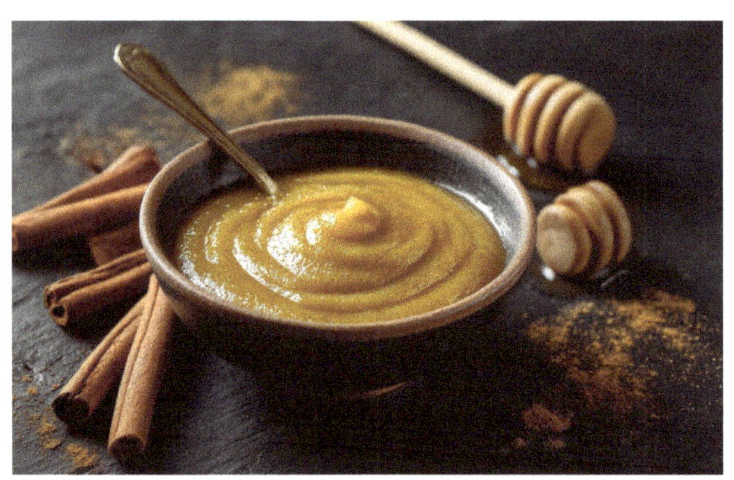

Why It Helps

Ashwagandha is an adaptogen that supports adrenal recovery and resilience.

How to Use

- Mix 2 tbsp ashwagandha powder with 4 tbsp raw honey.
- Take 1 tsp daily, stirred into warm milk.

Quick Remedy	Safety Notes	Variations
Stir ½ tsp into warm water if you're short on time.	Avoid if pregnant. Use cautiously with thyroid conditions.	Add cinnamon or cardamom for flavor and digestion.

7.   Chamomile & Lemon balm Foot Soak

Why It Helps

Chamomile soothes the nervous system and lemon balm eases anxious thoughts; a warm foot soak triggers whole-body relaxation.

How to Use

- ½ cup strong chamomile tea (4–6 tea bags) or ½ cup dried chamomile
- 1–2 tbsp dried lemon balm or a handful fresh leaves
- Pour infused/strained brew into a warm foot basin; soak 10–15 minutes.

Quick Remedy	Safety Notes	Variations
Add 10–15 drops chamomile tincture + 5–10 drops lemon balm tincture to a basin of warm tap water and soak 2–3 minutes.	Avoid if allergic to chamomile (Asteraceae). Tinctures contain alcohol; avoid for children or if you react to alcohol. Consult your clinician if you have diabetes, neuropathy, or open foot wounds.	Add ½ cup Epsom salts for extra muscle-relaxing support.

8. Skullcap Tea

Why It Helps

Skullcap calms irritability, overstimulation, and racing thoughts.

How to Use

- 1 tsp dried skullcap
- 1 cup hot water
  Steep 10 minutes, covered. Sip slowly.

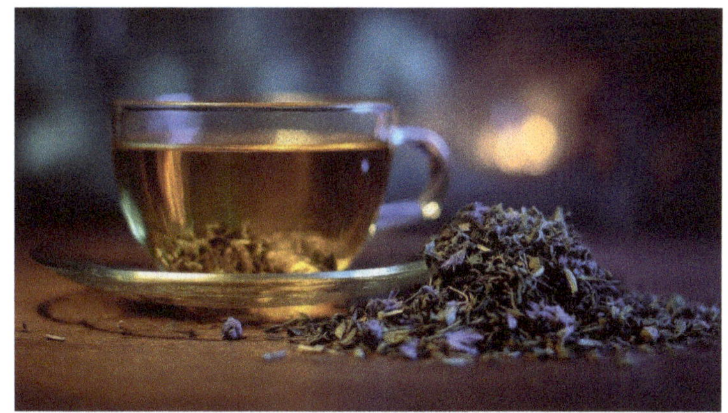

Quick Remedy	Safety Notes	Variations
Mix 30 drops tincture in water if you're short on time.	Avoid in pregnancy unless supervised.	Blend with chamomile for digestion + calm.

9. Passionflower & Valerian Blend

Why It Helps

Passionflower relaxes the mind; valerian relaxes the body. Together, they ease anxious insomnia.

How to Use

- Mix 30 drops passionflower tincture with 20 drops valerian tincture.
- Take 30 minutes before bed.

Quick Remedy	Safety Notes	Variations
Passionflower alone works well for daytime anxiety.	Valerian may cause grogginess. Avoid driving after use.	Try skullcap in place of valerian for lighter sedation.

10. Tulsi-Mint Afternoon Tea

Why It Helps

Tulsi lowers stress hormones, while peppermint refreshes and clears the mind.

How to Use

- 1 tsp dried tulsi
- 1 tsp dried peppermint
- 2 cups hot water
  Steep 10 minutes. Drink during afternoon slump.

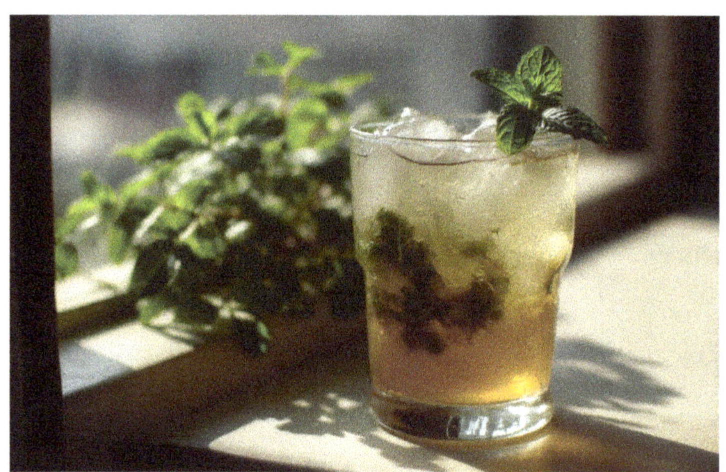

Quick Remedy	Safety Notes	Variations
Make a strong infusion and pour over ice for summer refreshment.	Safe for most; monitor if on blood thinners.	Add a slice of ginger for circulation.

Fatigue & Brain Fog Remedies (11–20)

11. Nettle Infusion for Steady Energy

Why It Helps

Nettles provide iron, calcium, magnesium, and chlorophyll, replenishing reserves that fatigue often depletes.

How to Use

- 1 oz dried nettle leaf
- 1 quart boiling water Steep 4–8 hours or overnight. Strain. Drink throughout the day.

Quick Remedy	Safety Notes	Variations
If short on time, steep 1 tbsp nettle in 1 cup hot water for 15 minutes.	Generally safe, though nettles can be mildly diuretic.	Add peppermint for freshness or lemon balm for calm energy.

12. Rosemary-Peppermint Tea

Why It Helps

Rosemary increases circulation and memory; peppermint refreshes and clears fog.

How to Use

- 1 tsp dried rosemary
- 1 tsp dried peppermint
- 1 cup hot water

  Steep 5 minutes. Drink warm.

Quick Remedy	Safety Notes	Variations
Chill a stronger brew and sip iced for afternoon clarity.	Avoid rosemary in medicinal doses during pregnancy.	Sweeten lightly with honey or add a slice of lemon.

13. Ashwagandha Night Milk

Why It Helps

Ashwagandha is an adaptogen that restores energy reserves and supports better sleep.

How to Use

- 1 tsp ashwagandha powder
- 1 cup milk (dairy or plant-based)
- ½ tsp cinnamon Simmer 5 minutes.

  Sweeten with honey. Drink before bed.

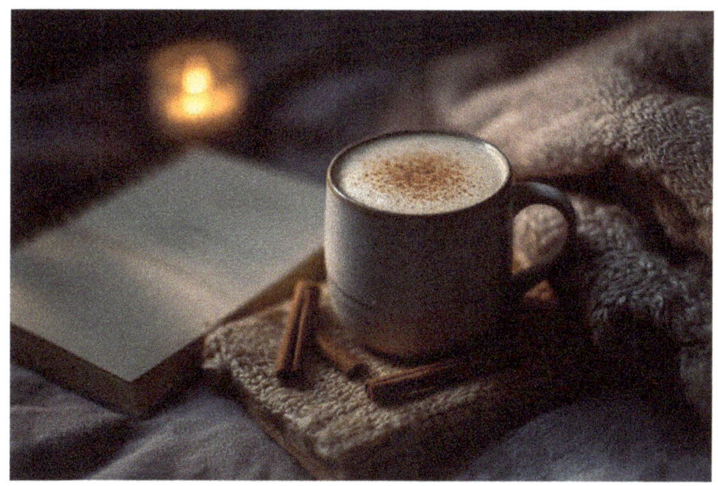

Quick Remedy	Safety Notes	Variations
Stir ½ tsp powder into warm milk when in a rush.	Avoid in pregnancy or if sensitive to nightshades.	Add nutmeg or cardamom for extra grounding.

14. Peppermint-Fennel Morning Tonic

Why It Helps

Peppermint gently awakens and soothes the stomach; fennel eases bloating and supports digestion. Warm water rehydrates after sleep.

How to Use

- 1 tsp fennel seeds, lightly crushed
- ½ tsp dried peppermint (or 5 fresh leaves)
- 1 cup warm water

  Steep 7–10 minutes. Drink on an empty stomach in the morning.

Quick Remedy	Safety Notes	Variations
Brew plain peppermint tea if fennel isn't on hand.	Peppermint may aggravate acid reflux; limit fennel to culinary amounts during pregnancy.	Add a pinch of cardamom or cinnamon for extra warmth.

15. Peppermint Oil Temple Rub

Why It Helps

Peppermint cools tension headaches and awakens the senses.

How to Use

- Dilute 2 drops peppermint essential oil in 1 tsp carrier oil
- Massage onto temples and back of neck

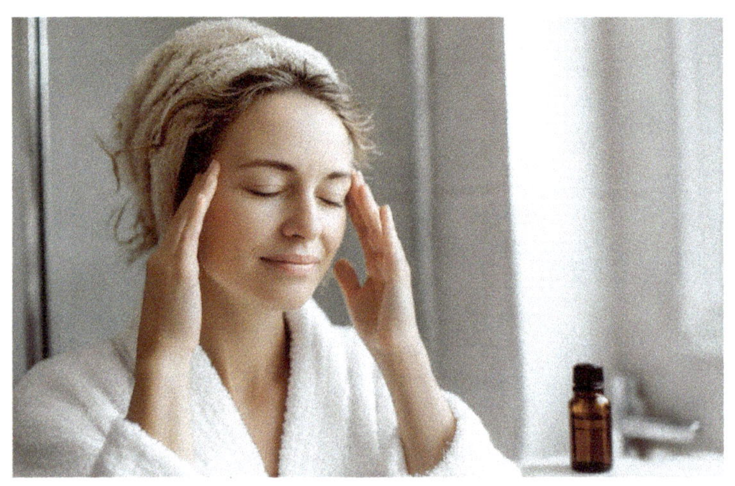

Quick Remedy	Safety Notes	Variations
Keep a pre-made roll-on bottle in your bag for instant relief.	Avoid near eyes; not for infants or very young children.	Blend with lavender oil for a calming twist.

16. Eleuthero (Siberian Ginseng) Tincture

Why It Helps

Eleuthero improves stamina, focus, and resilience to stress.

How to Use

- Take 30–40 drops tincture in water
- Use 2x daily for 4–6 weeks

Quick Remedy	Safety Notes	Variations
Pair with peppermint tea for an immediate lift while tincture works long term.	Avoid if you have uncontrolled hypertension.	Combine with ashwagandha for both day energy and night restoration.

17. Nettle & Peppermint Energy Tea

Why It Helps

Combines nettle's minerals with peppermint's freshness for a balanced lift.

How to Use

- 1 tbsp dried nettle
- 1 tsp dried peppermint
- 2 cups hot water

  Steep 15 minutes. Drink mid-morning.

Quick Remedy	Safety Notes	Variations
Steep 1 tsp of each for 5 minutes for a lighter brew.	Safe for most; monitor if taking diuretics.	Add lemon juice for brightness.

18. Rosemary Sniff Jar

Why It Helps

Inhaling rosemary boosts memory and alertness through scent pathways.

How to Use

- Fill a small jar with dried rosemary
- Open and inhale deeply for 30 seconds whenever fatigue strikes

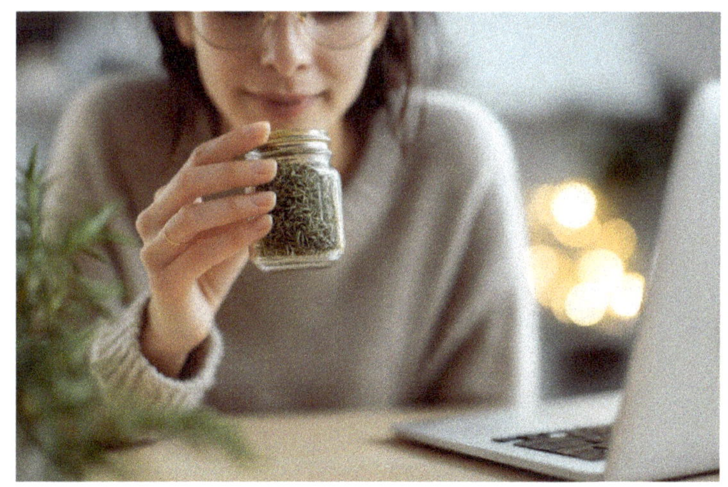

Quick Remedy	Safety Notes	Variations
Carry a sprig of fresh rosemary in your pocket for the same effect.	Avoid if strong scents trigger migraines.	Blend dried peppermint into the jar for extra lift.

19. Adaptogen Chai

Why It Helps

A warming blend of adaptogens and spices supports long-term energy.

How to Use

- 1 tsp ashwagandha root
- 1 tsp eleuthero root
- 1 cinnamon stick
- 2 slices fresh ginger
- 2 cups water + 1 cup milk

  Simmer 20 minutes. Strain and sweeten with honey.

Quick Remedy	Safety Notes	Variations
Make a simple spiced tea with ginger and cinnamon until adaptogens are on hand.	Avoid ashwagandha if pregnant; monitor caffeine sensitivity if adding black tea.	Add cardamom pods or cloves for a fuller chai flavor.

20. Peppermint & Licorice Afternoon Tea

Why It Helps

Peppermint refreshes; licorice root supports adrenal function.

How to Use

- 1 tsp dried peppermint
- ½ tsp dried licorice root
- 1 cup hot water

  Steep 10 minutes. Drink in the afternoon slump.

Quick Remedy	Safety Notes	Variations
Steep peppermint alone if licorice isn't available.	Avoid licorice if you have high blood pressure or are pregnant.	Add fennel seed for digestive comfort.

Sleep Remedies (21–30)

21. Chamomile Bedtime Tea

Why It Helps

Chamomile contains apigenin, a compound that binds to calming receptors in the brain, promoting relaxation and sleep.

How to Use

- 1 tsp dried chamomile flowers
- 1 cup hot water

    Steep 10 minutes, covered. Drink 30 minutes before bed.

Quick Remedy	Safety Notes	Variations
Use a chamomile tea bag if you're traveling or short on time.	Avoid if allergic to ragweed family plants.	Add honey and a slice of apple for a sweeter bedtime ritual.

22. Lavender Pillow Sachet

Why It Helps

Lavender's aroma has been shown in studies to reduce heart rate and promote deeper sleep.

How to Use

- Fill a small cloth sachet with dried lavender buds
- Squeeze sachet before bed to release oils
- Place near pillow

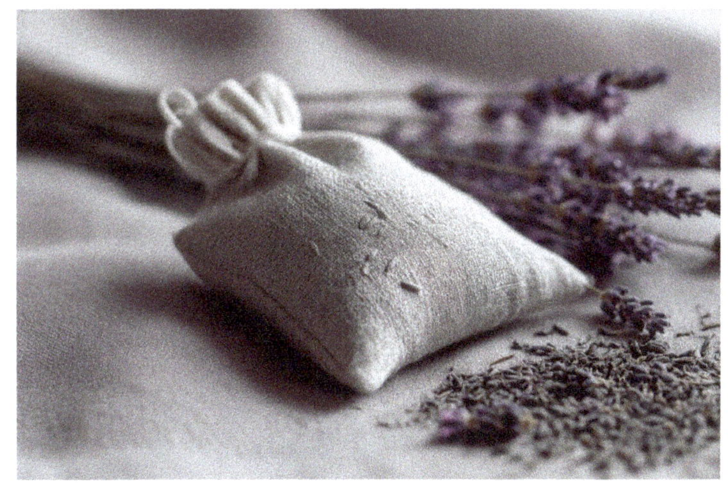

Quick Remedy	Safety Notes	Variations
Rub 1–2 drops lavender oil onto the corner of your pillow.	Avoid using strong essential oils directly on skin without dilution.	Combine with dried rose petals or hops for a floral blend.

23. Valerian Root Tincture

Why It Helps

Valerian relaxes muscles and supports deeper stages of sleep.

How to Use

- Take 30–40 drops valerian tincture in water 30 minutes before bed

Quick Remedy	Safety Notes	Variations
Combine with lemon balm tincture for extra calm.	May cause morning grogginess in some people. Avoid before driving.	Blend with passionflower for lighter sedation.

24. Passionflower Tea

Why It Helps

Passionflower quiets a racing mind and supports restful sleep.

How to Use

- 1 tsp dried passionflower
- 1 cup hot water

  Steep 10 minutes, covered. Drink at bedtime.

Quick Remedy	Safety Notes	Variations
Use tincture: 30 drops in water at night.	Avoid during pregnancy unless advised by a professional.	Add lemon balm or skullcap for stronger effect.

25. Warm Golden Milk

Why It Helps

Turmeric reduces inflammation; warm milk (dairy or plant-based) soothes the nervous system.

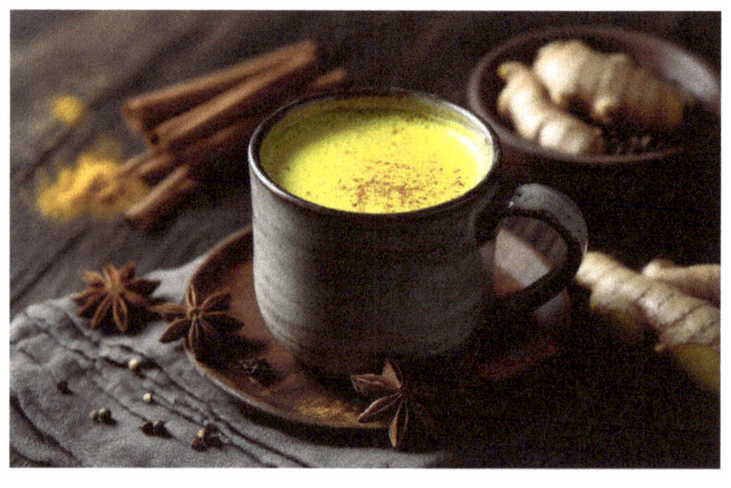

How to Use

- 1 cup milk
- ½ tsp turmeric powder
- Pinch black pepper

- ½ tsp cinnamon

  Simmer 5 minutes. Sweeten with honey. Drink warm before bed.

Quick Remedy	Safety Notes	Variations
Stir turmeric and cinnamon directly into warm milk.	Turmeric may interact with blood thinners; use with caution.	Add ½ tsp ashwagandha powder for deep repair.

26. Lemon Balm Evening Tea

Why It Helps

Lemon balm eases anxiety and tension, making sleep easier to reach.

How to Use

- 1 tsp dried lemon balm
- 1 cup hot water Steep 10 minutes. Drink an hour before bed.

Quick Remedy	Safety Notes	Variations
Take 30 drops tincture for faster results.	Not ideal for people with hypothyroidism in high doses.	Add lavender for extra calm.

27. Hops Sleep Sachet

Why It Helps

Hops contain natural sedative compounds that calm the nervous system.

How to Use

- Fill a cloth sachet with dried hops
- Place inside pillowcase at night

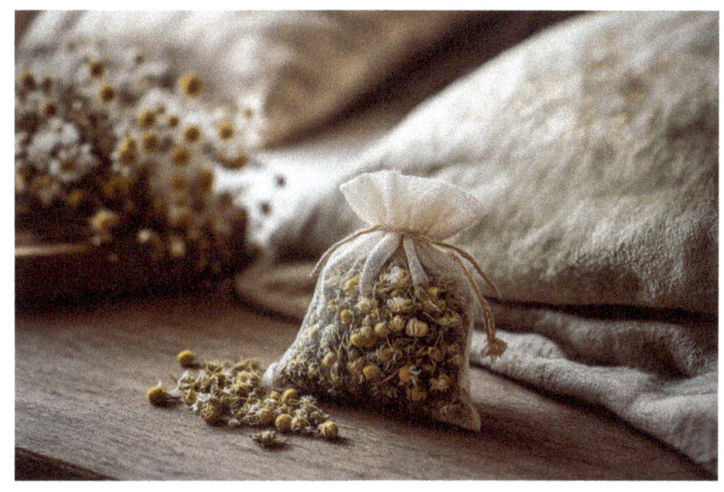

Quick Remedy	Safety Notes	Variations
Steep 1 tsp dried hops in tea if sachet isn't available.	Can be too strong for some; discontinue if it causes headaches.	Combine with lavender or chamomile in the sachet.

28. Skullcap Bedtime Tincture

Why It Helps

Skullcap relieves irritability and tension that interfere with sleep.

How to Use

- Take 30–40 drops tincture in water before bed

Quick Remedy	Safety Notes	Variations
Mix into chamomile tea for extra effect.	Avoid during pregnancy unless guided by a practitioner.	Blend with valerian for deeper sedation.

29. Oatstraw Night Infusion

Why It Helps

Oatstraw replenishes minerals that calm the nervous system and reduce nighttime restlessness.

How to Use

- 1 oz dried oatstraw

- 1 quart boiling water Steep 4–8 hours. Strain. Drink 1–2 cups in the evening.

Quick Remedy	Safety Notes	Variations
Steep 1 tbsp oatstraw in hot water for 15 minutes.	Avoid if allergic to oats.	Combine with chamomile or lemon balm for flavor and synergy.

30. Lavender Foot Soak

Why It Helps

Feet are rich in nerve endings; a soak signals the whole body to relax.

How to Use

- Add ½ cup dried lavender or 10 drops lavender oil to a basin of hot water.

- Soak feet for 15 minutes before bed.

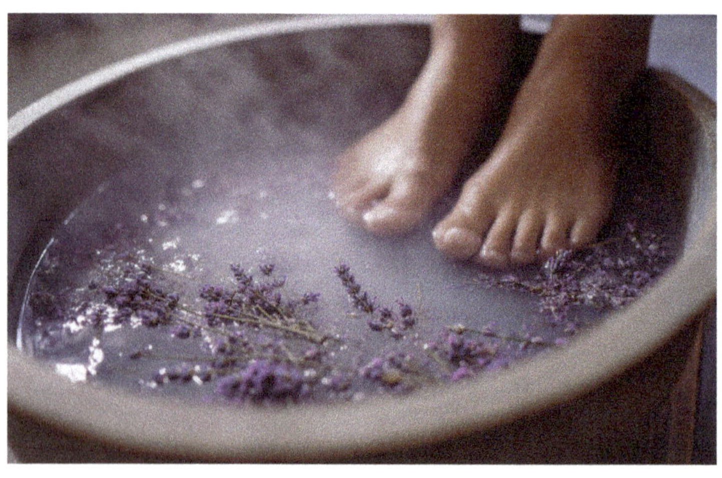

Quick Remedy	Safety Notes	Variations
Even a 5-minute soak before sleep is calming.	Ensure water is warm, not scalding.	Add ½ cup Epsom salts for extra magnesium support.

Immunity Remedies and Cold/Flu Preventatives (31–40)

31. Elderberry Syrup

Why It Helps

Elderberries are rich in flavonoids that support the immune system and reduce the severity of colds and flu.

How to Use

- 1 cup dried elderberries
- 4 cups water
- 1 cinnamon stick, 3 cloves, 1-inch ginger slice

  Simmer 45 minutes. Strain, then stir in 1 cup raw honey once cooled. Take 1 tsp daily for prevention or 1 tbsp every few hours if sick.

Quick Remedy	Safety Notes	Variations
Buy pre-made elderberry syrup for busy weeks.	Do not eat raw elderberries; they can cause nausea. Safe for children over 1 year when honey is included.	Add orange peel or echinacea root for stronger effect.

32. Garlic Honey

Why It Helps

Garlic contains allicin, a compound with antiviral and antibacterial properties. Honey soothes the throat.

How to Use

- Peel and lightly crush 6 garlic cloves
- Place in a small jar
- Cover with raw honey Let infuse 2–3 days. Take 1 tsp daily or at first sign of illness.

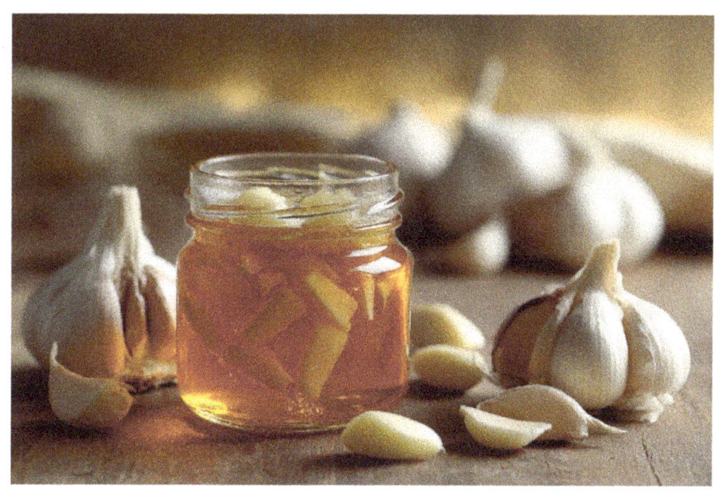

Quick Remedy	Safety Notes	Variations
Chew one raw clove at onset of symptoms if honey isn't prepared.	Raw garlic may irritate the stomach; eat with food.	Add ginger slices or cayenne pepper for extra kick.

33. Echinacea Tincture

Why It Helps

Echinacea stimulates immune cell activity and shortens the duration of colds when taken early.

How to Use

- Take 30–40 drops tincture in water every 2–3 hours at first sign of infection.
- Continue for 3–5 days.

Quick Remedy	Safety Notes	Variations
Add drops directly under the tongue for faster absorption.	Not for long-term daily use; best at onset of illness. Avoid if allergic to daisies.	Combine with elderberry syrup for dual action.

34. Fire Cider Tonic

Why It Helps

This traditional vinegar infusion clears sinuses and boosts immunity with antimicrobial herbs.

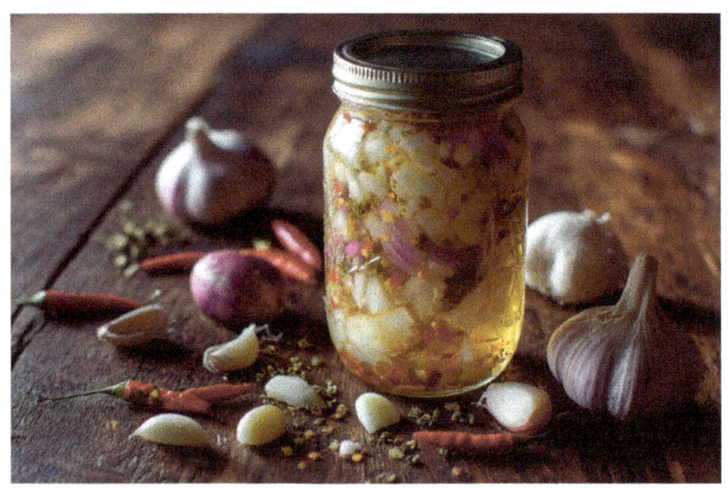

How to Use

- Fill a jar with chopped onion, garlic, ginger, horseradish, and hot peppers
- Cover with apple cider vinegar
- Steep 4 weeks, strain, and sweeten with honey Take 1 tbsp daily in winter or 1 tsp every few hours if sick.

Quick Remedy	Safety Notes	Variations
Add a splash of vinegar and honey to hot water with cayenne for a fast version.	May be too spicy for children or sensitive stomachs.	Add turmeric root or lemon slices for additional benefits.

35. Ginger Tea

Why It Helps

Ginger is warming, antimicrobial, and helps ease congestion while supporting digestion.

How to Use

- 1-inch slice fresh ginger root
- 1 cup hot water Simmer 10 minutes, strain, and drink hot.

Quick Remedy	Safety Notes	Variations
Chew fresh ginger slices or add powdered ginger to hot water.	Avoid large amounts if prone to acid reflux.	Add lemon and honey for soothing throat support.

36. Turmeric-Ginger Golden Paste

Why It Helps

Turmeric reduces inflammation while ginger boosts circulation and immune response.

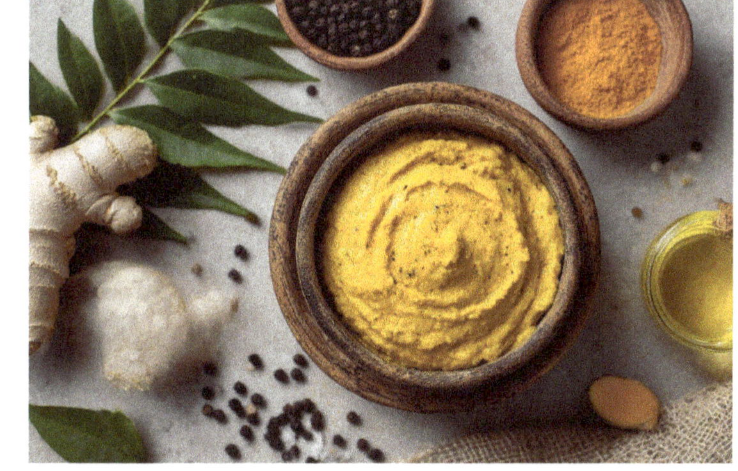

How to Use

- ¼ cup turmeric powder
- ½ cup water
- 2 tbsp grated ginger
- 2 tbsp coconut oil
- Pinch black pepper

  Simmer until thick. Store in fridge. Take ½ tsp daily stirred into warm milk or tea.

Quick Remedy	Safety Notes	Variations
Stir turmeric and ginger powder into warm milk with honey.	Turmeric may interact with blood thinners.	Add cinnamon or cardamom for flavor.

37. Elderflower Tea

Why It Helps

Elderflower reduces fever and clears congestion, especially during colds and flu.

How to Use

- 1 tsp dried elderflower
- 1 cup hot water Steep 10 minutes. Drink warm, 2–3 times daily.

Quick Remedy	Safety Notes	Variations
Use in steam inhalation by adding flowers to hot water and breathing vapors.	Avoid if allergic to elder plants.	Blend with peppermint and yarrow for classic fever tea.

38. Thyme Steam Inhalation

Why It Helps

Thyme is antimicrobial and helps clear respiratory congestion.

How to Use

- 2 tsp dried thyme
- 2 cups boiling water Pour into a bowl, lean over, cover head with a towel, and inhale for 5–10 minutes.

Quick Remedy	Safety Notes	Variations
Drink thyme tea (1 tsp in 1 cup hot water, steep 10 minutes).	Avoid steam burns by keeping face at a safe distance.	Add eucalyptus leaves or peppermint for stronger vapors.

39. Astragalus Broth

Why It Helps

Astragalus root strengthens long-term immunity and resilience.

How to Use

- Add 3–4 slices dried astragalus root to soups or broths
- Simmer for 1–2 hours, remove root before serving Enjoy weekly during cold season.

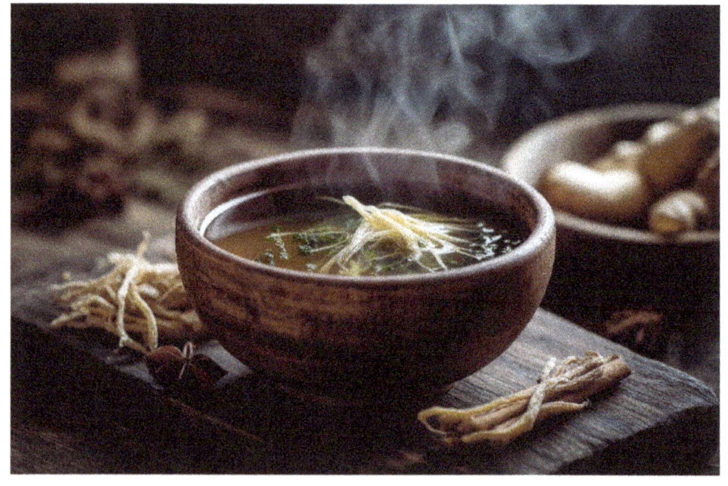

Quick Remedy	Safety Notes	Variations
Simmer astragalus root alone in water for 20 minutes for a tea.	Not for use during acute infection; best for prevention.	Pair with shiitake mushrooms for added immune support.

40. Lemon-Honey Drink

Why It Helps

Vitamin C from lemon and antibacterial properties of honey soothe sore throats and boost defenses.

How to Use

- Juice of ½ lemon
- 1 tbsp raw honey
- 1 cup warm water Stir and sip slowly.

Quick Remedy	Safety Notes	Variations
Mix lemon juice and honey directly on a spoon if water isn't available.	Do not give honey to children under 1 year.	Add grated ginger or a pinch of cayenne for stronger effect.

Quick Grab Box: Fastest Remedies

- **Lavender Hand Inhalation (Remedy 2):** 2 drops lavender essential oil in palms, inhale for 3 deep breaths. Relief in under a minute.

For Fatigue & Brain Fog

- **Rosemary Sniff Jar (Remedy 18):** Inhale deeply from a jar of dried rosemary or a fresh sprig. Mental clarity in 30 seconds.

For Sleep Struggles

- **Lavender Pillow Sachet (Remedy 22):** Squeeze sachet to release scent and place by your pillow. Calming effect begins as you breathe.

For Immunity

- **Garlic Honey (Remedy 32):** 1 tsp infused garlic honey daily or at first sign of a cold. Takes seconds to swallow, yet brings powerful support.

One of the most common worries I hear from beginners is: **"But what if I don't have time? What if I need relief right now?"**

The beauty of herbal medicine is that it can meet you exactly where you are. Some remedies do take time… a long infusion steeped overnight, a tincture built up in the body over weeks… but others work in minutes. These quick remedies are what I call my **"Grab & Go Apothecary."**

Think of them as the herbs you can lean on in the busiest of days, the moments when you don't have the luxury of brewing a pot of tea or simmering a syrup. These are the confidence-builders! The remedies that show you how immediate and powerful plants can be. The more you reach for them, the more second-nature herbalism becomes.

The Quick & Easy Grab & Go Apothecary

Here are the fastest remedies for each area we covered in this chapter:

Stress & Anxiety

Lavender Hand Inhalation (Remedy 2)

- Time to Prepare: 30 seconds.

- How it works: A single drop or two of lavender essential oil cupped in your palms shifts the nervous system almost instantly. Within a few breaths, your body begins to move from "fight or flight" into "rest and restore."

- Why it matters: Stress often arrives suddenly… during a difficult conversation, before a meeting, in a crowded grocery store. Having a remedy that works this fast is empowering. It proves to you that herbs are not just slow and subtle, they can act like lightning when used correctly.

Fatigue & Brain Fog

- Rosemary Sniff Jar (Remedy 18)

- Time to Prepare: 10 seconds (if the jar is already in your bag or desk drawer).

- How it works: Simply opening a jar of dried rosemary and inhaling deeply floods your senses with its sharp, piney aroma. Rosemary has been shown to improve memory, alertness, and circulation to the brain.

- Why it matters: When the mid-afternoon slump hits, most people reach for caffeine. But caffeine can overstimulate and leave you jittery. Rosemary offers clarity without the crash. It's also discreet and something you can do in a crowded space without drawing attention.

Sleep Struggles

Lavender Pillow Sachet (Remedy 22)

- Time to Prepare: Already ready-to-use…just keep it by your bed.

- How it works: Squeezing the sachet before bed releases aromatic oils that cue the body it's time to wind down. Lavender's calming effect on the nervous system is well documented! It encourages the release of calming neurotransmitters and slows a racing heart rate.

- Why it matters: Insomnia can feel overwhelming. But having something you can grab and use in seconds changes your relationship with bedtime. Even if sleep doesn't come right away, you're practicing a ritual that tells your body: *It's safe to rest.* Over time, this simple act creates a powerful sleep association.

Immunity

Garlic Honey (Remedy 32)

* Time to Prepare: If you've prepared a jar in advance, it's ready in under 5 seconds. Just open, scoop, and swallow a spoonful.

* How it works: Garlic is antimicrobial, antiviral, and stimulates the body's immune defenses. Honey adds soothing properties and carries garlic's potency smoothly into the body.

* Why it matters: The first tickle in the throat or ache in the body can leave you feeling helpless. But with garlic honey on hand, you have an immediate action step. This sense of empowerment—the knowledge that you can do something right now—is half the medicine.

Benefits of Herbal Remedies for Real-Life Relief:

* Build hands-on skill. You will learn how to measure drops, crush herbs, scoop honey… all tiny actions that build familiarity and confidence with new herbs and remedies!

* See tangible results. Herbs often work gently, but these remedies give you immediate feedback that keeps you motivated.

* Prevent overwhelm. Instead of waiting for the perfect moment to brew a long infusion, you'll know you can start small, today, in under a minute.

* Create new habits. Quick remedies are like steppingstones! They lead naturally into the deeper rituals and long-term practices.

A Final Encouragement

Start small. Keep your apothecary fresh. Use it. Notice what happens in your body. Write it down if you'd like. Let yourself be surprised at how much a sprig of rosemary, a spoonful of honey, or a single drop of lavender can shift your day.

REMEMBER: herbalism isn't about doing it all at once. It's about reaching for one small, doable thing and letting that be enough. Over time, those small things add up.

With these fast remedies at your fingertips, you're never without support. You can breathe easier, focus sharper, rest deeper, and feel stronger… starting right now.

Bonus Content

Scan the QR to download the **Quick Reference Guide**, a printable guide showing which herbs and rituals to use for sleep, stress, digestion, immunity, and more.

CHAPTER FIVE

Nature's Helpers Beyond Herbs

~Karla Wilson Baker

Healing isn't a single jar on a shelf. It's not a perfect morning routine you repeat without fail or a magic tincture that fixes everything in one night. Healing is a braid. It is the way you choose breakfast when you wake, the breath you take before you answer the difficult email, the bath you draw when your bones ache, the way you open the window for fresh air in winter and let the sea wind move through your home in summer. The herbs you learned in the last chapters are powerful threads in that braid. This chapter widens the weave.

When I was a child in Vermont, I thought my grandmother's medicine was the chamomile hanging from the rafters and the jars of yarrow and calendula lined up behind the flour. Years later, after I had moved to the Oregon coast and had two children of my own, I understood that her medicine was

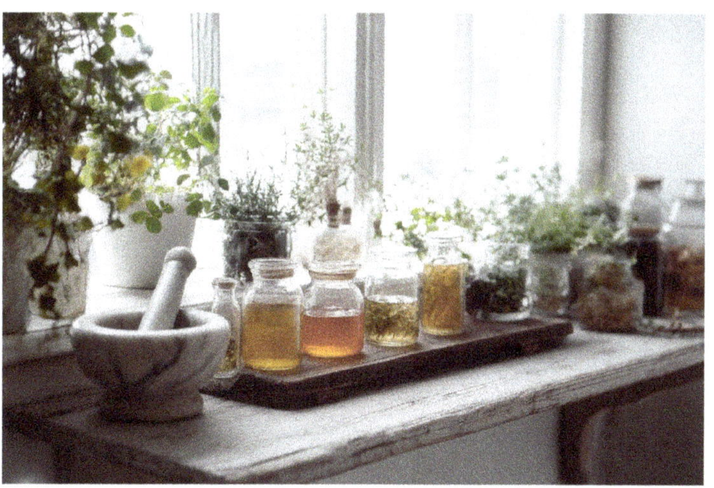

everywhere. It was in the pots of soup simmering low all afternoon. It was in the crock of sauerkraut quietly fizzing in a corner of the pantry. It was in the way she mindfully rinsed her hands with cool water after weeding and then pressed a rose petal to her wrist and breathed. It was in the way she believed that a home should smell like fresh air, wood smoke, and dinner, not chemicals. Her medicine was alive inside her life.

This chapter is for that kind of medicine. We will keep to the same promise of practicality you have seen throughout this book. Everything here is meant to fit into a real day with a real budget in a small kitchen. You won't need special equipment. You won't need to turn your apartment into a spa. You'll need only attention and a willingness to begin. Think of these as your helpers beyond the herb jars: healing foods, flower essences, essential oils and aromatics, baths and breathwork, and a handful of clean-living swaps that lower the burden on your body without draining your wallet.

You will notice that I'm not asking you to do all seventeen at once. Choose one or two. Let them become familiar. When you feel their goodness, choose another. This is how we build a life that heals us while we live it.

Healing Foods: Everyday Medicine You Already Eat

(Remedies 1–6)

Remedy 1. Fermented Foods for a Happier Gut

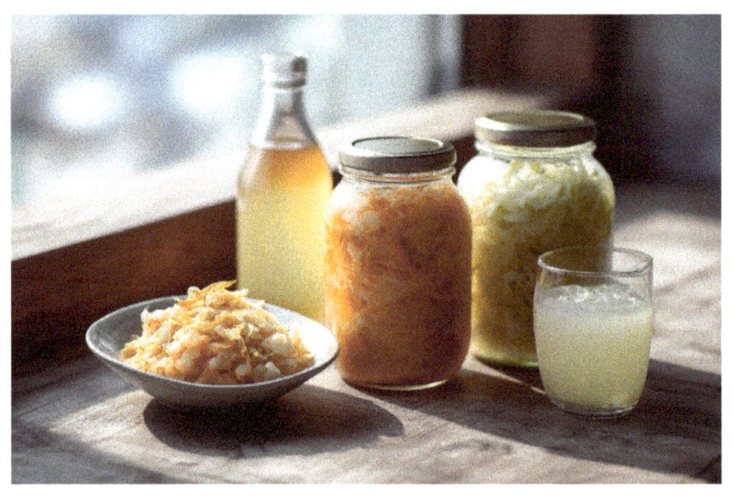

What it is: Living foods like sauerkraut, kimchi, kefir, plain yogurt with live cultures, and kombucha bring beneficial bacteria into the digestive tract and help the community of microbes in your gut become more diverse and resilient. A more resilient gut often means calmer digestion, steadier immunity, and even a brighter mood.

How to use: start small. If you are new to ferments, add one forkful of sauerkraut to lunch or dinner. Sip half a cup of kefir or kombucha. Repeat most days for three weeks. The benefits come from consistency. If your digestion is sensitive, begin with a teaspoon and build slowly.

How to Use

- Eat 1–2 forkfuls sauerkraut, kimchi, or other raw ferments daily.
- Drink ½ cup kefir or kombucha.
- Consistency is key—start small if new to ferments.

Quick Remedy	Safety Notes	Variations
Buy live-culture ferments at the store if you don't have time to make your own.	If you're new to ferments, start with a teaspoon daily to avoid bloating. Safety: If a ferment smells rotten or grows fuzzy mold on top, compost it and start again. A tangy, pleasantly sour smell is what you want.	Try pickled carrots with ginger or beet kvass for different flavors. In winter, I like a simple carrot and ginger kraut with fish or beans. In summer, I spoon kimchi on rice with a fried egg and herbs from the windowsill. If dairy isn't your friend, choose water kefir, kombucha, kraut, or kimchi.

Budget and sourcing: Store-bought is fine if the label says live cultures and the jar is in the refrigerated section. If you want to make your own, you need only cabbage, salt, and a jar. Cabbage plus salt becomes lively medicine with time.

LYDIA'S NOTE: The first winter I kept a crock again, the house felt different. There was a quiet pulse on the counter, a sense that something alive was happening in the kitchen even when the garden slept.

Remedy 2. Bone Broth or Mineral Broth for Deep Repair

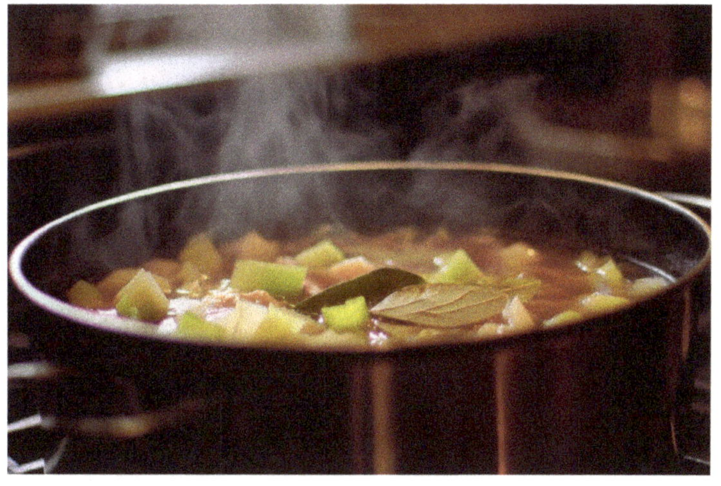

What it is: A slow-simmered stock that extracts collagen, minerals, and soothing amino acids from bones and connective tissue. If you prefer plants, a mineral broth made from seaweed, mushrooms, onion, celery, carrot, and parsley brings similar nourishment.

How to use: Place leftover roasted chicken bones or two pounds of marrow and knuckle bones in a pot with onion, carrot, celery, garlic, a bay leaf, a splash of vinegar, and water to cover. Simmer at the gentlest bubble for eight to twelve hours. Strain. Sip warm with a pinch of sea salt, or use as the base for soups and grains. For a plant version, simmer kombu, dried shiitake or reishi, onion, carrot, celery, parsley stems, and peppercorns for two to four hours and strain.

How to Use

- **Bone broth:** Simmer 2 lbs. bones with onion, carrot, celery, garlic, 1 tbsp vinegar, and water 8–12 hours. Strain.
- **Mineral broth:** Simmer 1 kombu strip, 2 dried shiitake mushrooms, onion, carrot, celery, and parsley stems 2–4 hours. Strain.

Sip 1 cup daily or use as soup base.

Quick Remedy	Safety Notes	Variations
Simmer vegetables and kombu 30 minutes for a lighter mineral tea.	If on a low-sodium diet, season lightly.	Add fresh ginger and turmeric for an immune boost. Add slices of ginger and a stick of cinnamon when you are run down. Add nettle leaves in the last hour for a green mineral lift. If you're on a very low-sodium diet, season lightly and discuss routine use with your clinician.

Remedy 3. Omega-3s From Flax, Chia, or Fatty Fish

What it is: Anti-inflammatory fats that support brain health, mood, hormones, and skin.

How to use: Stir a tablespoon of freshly ground flaxseed into oatmeal or smoothies. Soak a tablespoon of chia seeds in water for fifteen minutes and add to yogurt with berries. Eat salmon or sardines two to three times a week. If you choose a capsule, look for products that provide both EPA and DHA.

How to Use

- Stir 1 tbsp ground flaxseed or chia into oatmeal or smoothies daily.
- Eat salmon, sardines, or mackerel 2–3 times weekly.

Quick Remedy	Safety Notes	Variations
Take 1 tsp flaxseed oil straight from a spoon.	Buy flax whole and grind fresh to prevent rancidity.	Sprinkle walnuts or hemp seeds over salads for extra omega-3s. Toasted walnuts and pumpkin seeds on salads, tahini in dressings, and a drizzle of olive oil at the table also support a better fat balance

Budget and sourcing note: Canned wild salmon and sardines are often affordable and keep in the cupboard. Buy whole flax and grind small amounts each week so it stays fresh.

Remedy 4. Seasonal Bitter Greens for Liver and Mood

What it is: Dandelion greens in spring, arugula in summer, chicory in autumn, and kale or collards in winter. Bitter greens wake the digestive organs, encourage bile flow, and can lift a heavy mood that comes from sluggish digestion.

How to use: Add a handful of raw bitter greens to your plate at lunch and dinner. Dress with lemon and olive oil. If raw greens trouble you, sauté with garlic in olive oil until tender. Two small servings a day is plenty.

How to Use

- Eat 1 handful fresh dandelion, arugula, chicory, or kale daily.
- Toss with lemon juice and olive oil, or sauté lightly with garlic.

Quick Remedy	Safety Notes	Variations
Steep 1 tsp dried dandelion leaf in 1 cup hot water for a simple bitter tonic.	Use cautiously if you have gallbladder disease—start with small amounts.	Mix with sweet greens like spinach for a milder taste.

5. Garlic & Onion Habit

Why It Helps

Garlic and onions contain sulfur compounds with antimicrobial and circulatory benefits. Regular use reduces risk of infections and supports detoxification.

How to Use

- Add 1 clove raw or cooked garlic to daily meals.
- Sauté onion in olive oil as a base for soups and grains.

Quick Remedy	Safety Notes	Variations
Crush a clove of garlic and swallow with honey at first sign of illness.	Raw garlic may upset sensitive stomachs, cook gently if needed. If you take bile duct medications or have gallbladder disease, start with very small servings and notice how you feel.	Roast garlic and spread on bread for a mellow, sweet remedy. In spring, toss dandelion greens with sliced radish and boiled eggs. In winter, braise kale with onion and a splash of apple cider vinegar.

LYDIA'S NOTE: I keep a bowl washed and ready in the fridge. When the greens are within reach, I actually eat them.

Remedy 5. The Garlic and Onion Habit

What it is: A daily practice of cooking with alliums. Garlic and onions contain sulfur compounds that support detoxification pathways and have broad antimicrobial effects. They keep your kitchen fragrant and your meals satisfying.

How to use: Sauté a sliced onion in olive oil as the first step in soups, sauces, and beans. Smash a clove of garlic and add it near the end of cooking or whisk it into lemon juice and olive oil for a simple dressing. Aim for some version, raw or cooked, most days.

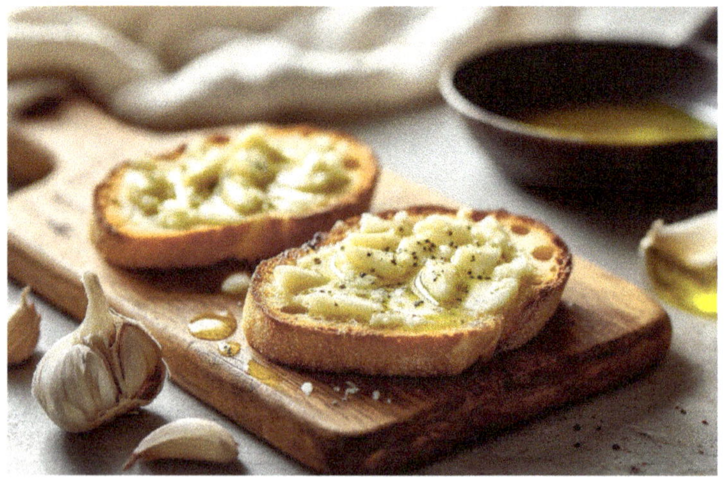

Variations	Safety
Try roasted garlic spread on warm toast with a drizzle of olive oil and a pinch of sea salt when you are coming down with something.	Raw garlic can irritate a sensitive stomach. If that is you, cook it gently or use small amounts.

Remedy 6. Sea Vegetables for Thyroid and Minerals

What it is: Nori, kelp, dulse, and wakame. These sea plants concentrate iodine and trace minerals that can be scarce inland.

How to use: Slip a strip of kombu into pots of beans or broth. Crumble dulse over salads and eggs. Roll rice and vegetables in nori sheets for simple hand rolls.

Budget and sourcing: A single bag of kombu or dulse flakes lasts a long time. Keep it dry in a jar. Even one pinch a day adds up.

Safety
If you have a thyroid condition, use seaweed sparingly at first, and consult your practitioner about routine iodine intake.

Flower Essences & Emotional Remedies (Remedies 7–9)

7. Rescue Remedy

Why It Helps

A blend of five Bach flower essences, Rescue Remedy is famous for easing acute stress, shock, or grief. It works subtly on the emotional body, helping restore balance.

How to Use

- Place 4 drops under the tongue or in 1 cup water
- Repeat up to 3 times daily during stressful events

Quick Remedy	Safety Notes	Variations
Carry a small bottle in your bag and use before difficult conversations, flights, or exams.	Contains a small amount of alcohol as preservative. If sensitive, dilute in hot water and let sit before drinking.	Available as spray or lozenges for travel.

8. Rose Essence

Why It Helps

Rose essence gently opens and soothes the heart, easing grief, heartbreak, or emotional fatigue.

How to Use

- Take 4 drops under the tongue or in water
- Use daily for 2–3 weeks during emotional heaviness

Quick Remedy	Safety Notes	Variations
Add a few drops to a cup of tea before a stressful interaction.	Safe for most people, including children.	Pair with Rescue Remedy for greater comfort during loss or transition.

9. Wild Oat Essence

Why It Helps

Wild oat essence is used for times of confusion, lack of direction, or life transitions. It helps bring clarity and alignment with purpose.

How to Use

- Take 4 drops under the tongue, 2–4 times daily
- Continue for several weeks while journaling or reflecting

Quick Remedy	Safety Notes	Variations
Add to a morning glass of water as a daily ritual during career or life changes.	Contains alcohol as preservative; dilute in warm water if avoiding.	Combine with gentian for courage or hornbeam for motivation.

Essential Oils & Aromatic Helpers (Remedies 10–12)

10. Citrus Diffusion

Why It Helps

Citrus oils like orange, grapefruit, and lemon uplift mood and improve focus. Studies show they can reduce anxiety and boost alertness.

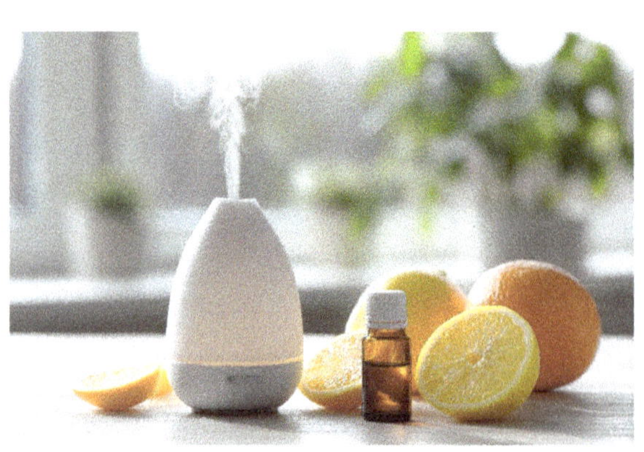

How to Use

- Add 4–5 drops citrus oil to a diffuser filled with water
- Run in morning or early afternoon

Quick Remedy	Safety Notes	Variations
Place 1 drop on a cotton ball and keep near workspace.	Citrus oils can cause photosensitivity if applied to skin—avoid sun exposure after topical use.	Blend with lavender for calm or rosemary for sharper focus.

11. Peppermint Roll-On

Why It Helps

Peppermint oil cools, relieves headaches, and improves alertness.

How to Use

- Dilute 2–3 drops peppermint oil in 1 tsp carrier oil
- Apply to temples, back of neck, or wrists

Quick Remedy	Safety Notes	Variations
Keep a pre-made roll-on in your bag for headaches or fatigue.	Avoid near eyes. Not for infants or small children.	Blend with lavender oil for both relaxation and relief.

12. Frankincense for Meditation

Why It Helps

Frankincense deepens the breath, calms the nervous system, and supports meditation. Its aroma has been used in sacred practices for centuries.

How to Use

- Place 1 drop in palms, rub together, inhale deeply
- Diffuse 4–5 drops in the evening during quiet time

Quick Remedy	Safety Notes	Variations
Add 1 drop to a bowl of hot water, cover head with towel, and inhale for a few breaths.	Strong aroma—introduce slowly if sensitive.	Blend with sandalwood or myrrh for grounding rituals.

Baths, Breath, & Body Rituals (Remedies 13–15)

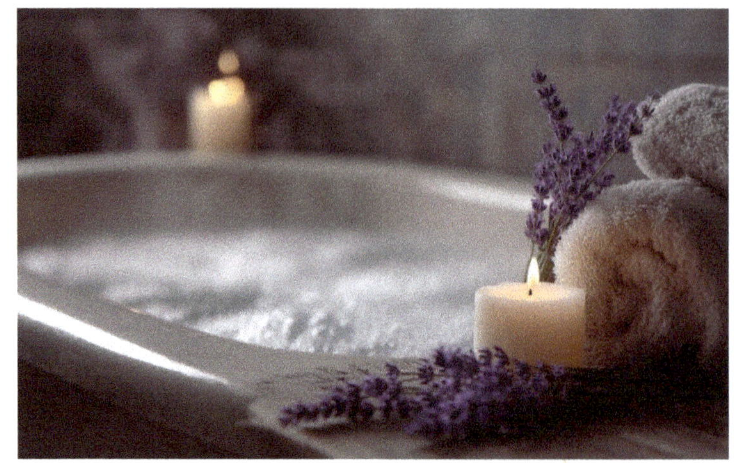

13. Evening Epsom Salt Bath

Why It Helps

Epsom salts provide magnesium, which relaxes muscles and reduces stress. Warm water improves circulation and calms the nervous system.

How to Use

- Add 1 cup Epsom salts to a warm bath
- Soak 20 minutes before bed

Quick Remedy	Safety Notes	Variations
Use a foot soak with ½ cup salts if no tub.	Avoid very hot water if you have high blood pressure.	Add 10 drops lavender oil for extra relaxation.

14. 4–7–8 Breath

Why It Helps

This breathing pattern lowers heart rate and activates the parasympathetic nervous system.

How to Use

- Inhale through nose for 4 counts
- Hold for 7 counts
- Exhale through mouth for 8 counts
- Repeat 3–4 rounds

Quick Remedy	Safety Notes	Variations
Use anywhere—in the car, at your desk, before bed.	If holding breath feels uncomfortable, shorten counts but keep the ratio.	Pair with aromatherapy by inhaling lavender or citrus while breathing.

15. Castor Oil Pack

Why It Helps

Castor oil increases circulation, supports liver function, and eases cramps.

How to Use

- Soak cotton flannel in castor oil
- Place on abdomen, cover with wrap or towel
- Add hot water bottle, rest 30–60 minutes

Quick Remedy	Safety Notes	Variations
Apply for 20 minutes during menstrual cramps.	Avoid during pregnancy. Do not apply to broken skin.	Use over liver in winter for gentle detox support.

Clean Living Swaps (Remedies 16–17)

16. Vinegar & Baking Soda Cleaners

Why It Helps

Homemade cleaners reduce chemical load, protect lungs, and save money. Vinegar is antibacterial; baking soda scrubs effectively.

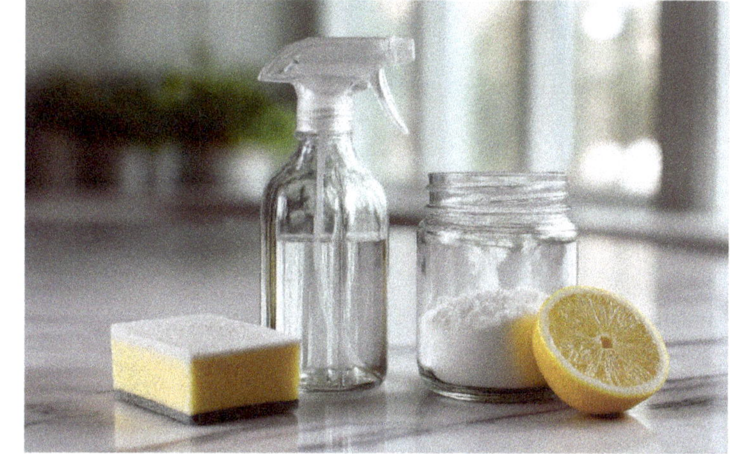

How to Use

- Mix 1 part vinegar to 1 part water in a spray bottle
- Add a few drops essential oil if desired
- Use baking soda for scrubbing sinks or tubs

Quick Remedy	Safety Notes	Variations
Wipe counters with diluted vinegar water.	Never mix vinegar with bleach.	Infuse vinegar with citrus peels for a fresher scent.

17. Natural Body Care Swaps

Why It Helps

Many body products contain harsh chemicals. Replacing them lowers toxic exposure and supports skin health.

How to Use

- Replace moisturizer with coconut oil or shea butter
- Use castile soap diluted for hand/body wash
- Try oil cleansing for the face

Quick Remedy	Safety Notes	Variations
Rub coconut oil onto dry skin in seconds.	Always patch test new products.	Make small swaps—start with soap or lotion, then move on to shampoo or deodorant.

Weaving It into a Day

I promised that you wouldn't need extra hours. Let me show you how this can look inside an ordinary Tuesday.

You wake up, open the window for a minute and breathe the cool air. While the kettle heats, you splash your face and take four slow breaths in the 4–7–8 rhythm. Breakfast is a bowl of warm oats scattered with walnuts and a spoon of ground flax, not because you're perfect but because the flax jar sits right next to the tea. You put a small bowl of sauerkraut on the table and spoon a little onto your plate. You don't announce it as medicine. You just eat.

Before your first meeting, you place a drop of sweet orange onto a cotton ball near your keyboard. When your shoulders creep toward your ears near midafternoon, you roll peppermint across the base of your skull and rub the extra into your palms to inhale. Dinner is simple soup made from last weekend's broth with beans and chopped kale. After dishes, you spray the counters with your vinegar cleaner and put the bottle back under the sink. An hour later, you pour a bath, add Epsom salts, and read three pages. Just before bed, you squeeze the lavender sachet at your pillow and breathe the softer air.

This is how your day weaves in these remedies. It's not heroic. It's a series of small decisions that keep you near yourself in a devotional way. Over weeks, these choices change your body gently. Your digestion steadies. Your sleep deepens. Your shoulders live an inch lower. Your home feels friendlier to breathe in. You start to trust not just the jars on your shelf but your own hands.

Bringing The Helpers Together

You now have seventeen helpers that belong to the life you already live. Some sit quietly on the counter, some fizz in a jar, some ride in your pocket, some give off scent like a breeze. They are strong enough to matter and simple enough to use. They ask you to notice what you already do and to turn those motions slightly toward healing.

If you need a place to begin, choose three. A food, a feeling, and a ritual. For food, perhaps a forkful of kraut at lunch or a strip of kombu in your soup. For feeling, perhaps rose essence when your heart pinches. For ritual, perhaps a bath with Epsom salts on Sunday night. Let those be your beginning. When they are easy, add a cleaner under the sink that doesn't make you cough, a citrus cotton ball at the desk, a roller bottle for the car. Let the helpers arrive like guests and then become family.

I have learned that the body responds with gratitude when you lower its burden and feed it well. The changes don't shout. They add up. The next cold is simpler. The next deadline doesn't tangle your breath. The next winter, your skin is steadier because you remembered the broth pot!

Action Steps

Choose one helper from each group and use them this week. Choose a fermented food or a broth. Choose a flower essence for your current mood. Choose one aromatic practice for morning or evening. Choose one bath or breath ritual. Choose one household or body-care swap. Write one line each night about how you felt. The point is not perfection. The point is practice.

You're not adding chores to your life. You're letting your life be the medicine.

CHAPTER SIX

Women's Wellness in a Modern World

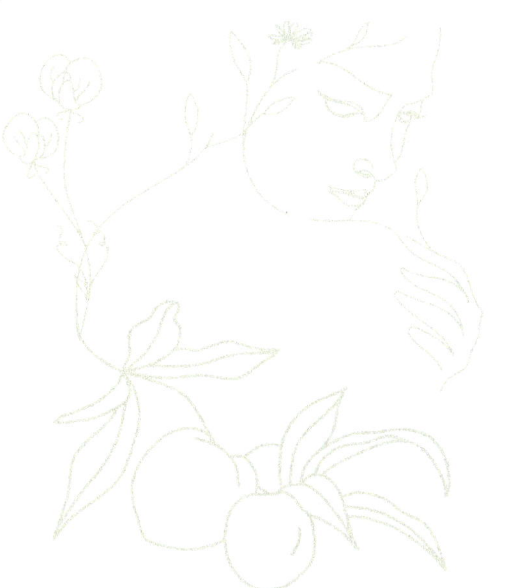

> "The rhythm of a woman's body is not a flaw to be managed. It is a compass to be listened to, a tide that carries wisdom with every rise and fall."
>
> — *Lydia Rosemont*

When I look back on my own healing, one of the biggest shifts came when I stopped fighting my body's rhythms and started listening to them. In my late thirties, after two children and years of carrying too much, I realized that stress, exhaustion, and mood swings weren't signs that my body was failing. They were signals. My body was speaking and asking for more support, nourishment, and slowness. I just needed to learn her language.

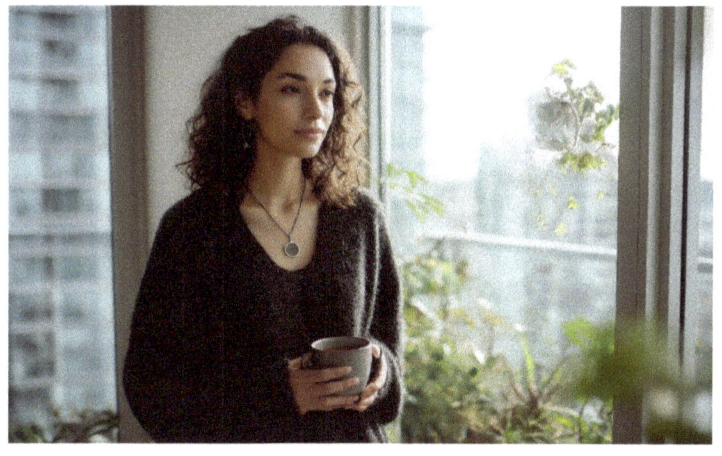

For women today, this language is harder to hear. We live in a masculine culture that often demands we push through: through PMS, through cramps, through perimenopause hot flashes, through the fog of caregiving or professional pressure. We are asked to give endlessly without pausing to refill. Many of us feel like "superwomen" and "girl bosses"—capable, yes, but running on fumes.

This chapter is about reclaiming wellness for women in a modern world. Herbs and natural practices can offer real support for hormonal balance, for cyclical nourishment, and for sustaining energy in the roles we hold. The remedies here are simple, targeted, and designed to fit into busy lives. My hope is that you feel recognized, supported, and equipped with tools that remind you: you are not broken. You are whole, and your wellness can flourish with care, slowness, and gentle tending.

Hormonal Harmony (Remedies 1–5)

Hormones shape so much of a woman's life! Energy, mood, skin, digestion, and even sleep directly influence your hormones. When they flow smoothly, we feel balanced. When they are disrupted, we feel it everywhere. The following remedies focus on common challenges like PMS, perimenopause, and emotional swings.

1. Vitex Berry Tea for Cycle Regularity

Why It Helps

Vitex (chaste tree berry) gently supports the pituitary gland, helping balance estrogen and progesterone. It is especially helpful for PMS and irregular cycles.

How to Use

- 1 tsp crushed vitex berries
- 1 cup hot water

    Steep 10 minutes, covered. Drink each morning.

Quick Remedy	Safety Notes	Variations
Vitex tincture: 30–40 drops in water once daily.	Not recommended during pregnancy. Give vitex at least three months for full effect.	Blend with lemon balm for added stress relief.

2. Cramp Bark Tincture for Menstrual Pain

Why It Helps

Cramp bark relaxes uterine muscles, easing spasms and painful cramps.

How to Use

- Take 30–40 drops tincture in water
- Repeat every 3–4 hours as needed during cramps

Quick Remedy	Safety Notes	Variations
Combine with ginger tea for faster relief and warmth.	Safe for short-term use; avoid exceeding recommended doses.	Substitute with black haw tincture if cramp bark isn't available.

3. Maca Root Powder for Perimenopause Energy

Why It Helps

Maca supports hormone balance, improves stamina, and helps with mood swings during perimenopause.

How to Use

- Add 1–2 tsp maca powder to smoothies, oatmeal, or yogurt daily

Quick Remedy	Safety Notes	Variations
Mix 1 tsp maca powder in warm milk with honey.	May be too stimulating for some—start with small amounts. Avoid if pregnant.	Pair with cacao powder for a mocha-like energizing blend.

4. Seed Cycling for Hormone Balance

Why It Helps

Specific seeds provide lignans, minerals, and fatty acids that gently support hormonal fluctuations through the menstrual cycle.

How to Use

- Days 1–14: 1 tbsp flax + 1 tbsp pumpkin seeds daily
- Days 15–28: 1 tbsp sesame + 1 tbsp sunflower seeds daily

  Eat ground or whole, sprinkled on salads, yogurt, or smoothies.

Quick Remedy	Safety Notes	Variations
Add mixed seed butter (like tahini or sunflower butter) to toast if short on time.	Safe for most people; seeds are gentle and food-based.	If you don't track cycles, simply rotate seeds weekly.

5. Sage Tea for Hot Flashes

Why It Helps

Sage helps regulate sweating and temperature, easing hot flashes and night sweats common in perimenopause and menopause.

How to Use

- 1 tsp dried sage
- 1 cup hot water Steep 10 minutes. Drink once daily or during hot flash episodes.

Quick Remedy	Safety Notes	Variations
Take 20–30 drops sage tincture in water for faster effect.	Avoid medicinal doses during pregnancy or breastfeeding.	Blend with peppermint for a cooling, refreshing tea.

Nourishing Your Cycle & Nervous System (Remedies 6–10)

A woman's cycle isn't just hormonal, it's deeply tied to the nervous system. Stress can shorten, lengthen, or even pause menstruation. Nourishing both body and nerves is key.

6. Raspberry Leaf Tea for Tone & Strength

Why It Helps

Raspberry leaf is a uterine tonic, easing heavy periods and supporting menstrual health.

How to Use

- 1 tbsp dried raspberry leaf
- 1 cup hot water Steep 10–15 minutes. Drink once or twice daily.

Quick Remedy	Safety Notes	Variations
Use a tea bag for convenience.	Safe for most; avoid in early pregnancy unless guided by a midwife.	Combine with nettle for added mineral support.

7. Chamomile Compress for PMS Bloating

Why It Helps

Chamomile relaxes muscles and reduces bloating when applied externally.

How to Use

- Brew 2 tbsp dried chamomile in 2 cups hot water for 10 minutes
- Soak cloth, wring gently, and place over abdomen for 15 minutes

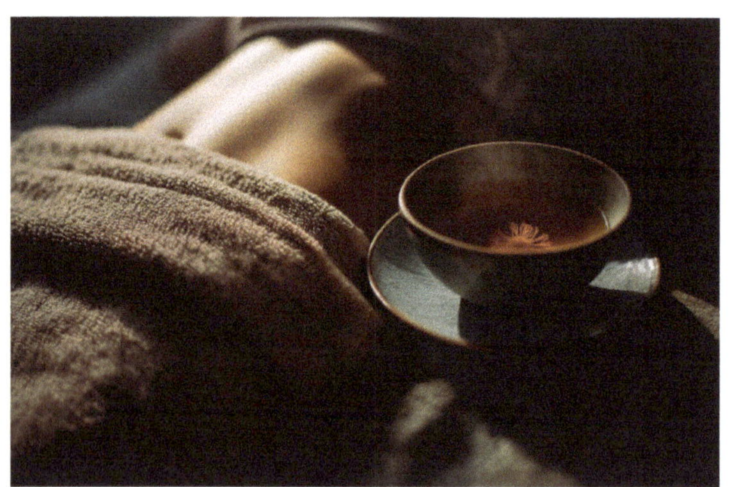

Quick Remedy	Safety Notes	Variations
Microwave a damp washcloth for 20 seconds and add 2 drops chamomile oil.	Avoid if allergic to ragweed family plants.	Add lavender oil to the compress for relaxation.

8. Oatstraw Infusion for Nerve Nourishment

Why It Helps

Oatstraw is rich in minerals, rebuilding resilience and calming the nervous system.

How to Use

- 1 oz dried oatstraw

- 1 quart boiling water

  Steep 4–8 hours or overnight. Drink throughout the day.

Quick Remedy	Safety Notes	Variations
Steep 1 tbsp oatstraw in hot water for 15 minutes.	Avoid if allergic to oats.	Blend with lemon balm for extra calm.

9. Magnesium-Rich Evening Snack

Why It Helps

Magnesium eases cramps, reduces PMS mood swings, and improves sleep.

How to Use

- Eat 1 oz pumpkin seeds, almonds, or dark chocolate in the evening

Quick Remedy	Safety Notes	Variations
Dissolve 1 tsp magnesium powder in water before bed.	Excess magnesium may cause loose stools—adjust dose as needed.	Sprinkle pumpkin seeds over salads or yogurt.

10. Lavender Foot Soak for Emotional Release

Why It Helps

Warm water and lavender oil relax the nervous system, easing tension.

How to Use

- Add ½ cup Epsom salts + 8 drops lavender oil to a basin of warm water
- Soak feet 15 minutes during PMS or stressful days

Quick Remedy	Safety Notes	Variations
Add 2 drops lavender oil to a damp washcloth and inhale deeply.	Avoid very hot water for those with circulation issues.	Add rose petals for a heart-soothing effect.

Energy Rituals for Busy Women (Remedies 11–15)

Many women juggle careers, caregiving, and community roles. Energy rituals prevent burnout and remind us we are not machines.

11. Nettle & Peppermint Tea for Steady Energy

Why It Helps

Nettle's minerals and peppermint's freshness support energy without caffeine crashes.

How to Use

- 1 tbsp dried nettle
- 1 tsp dried peppermint
- 2 cups hot water
  Steep 15 minutes. Drink mid-morning.

Quick Remedy	Safety Notes	Variations
Steep 1 tsp of each for 5 minutes.	Mildly diuretic; stay hydrated.	Add lemon juice for brightness.

12. Rosemary Inhalation Before Meetings

Why It Helps

Rosemary sharpens focus and memory.

How to Use

- Rub fresh rosemary sprig or dried leaves between fingers
- Inhale deeply for 30 seconds

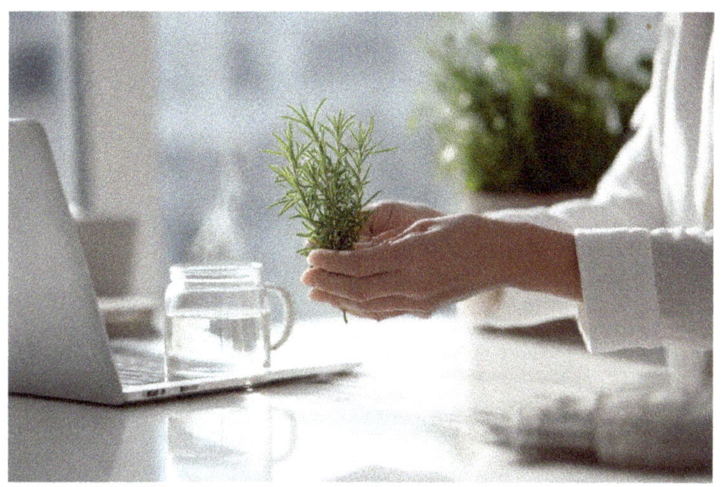

Quick Remedy	Safety Notes	Variations
Carry a small jar of dried rosemary in your bag.	Avoid strong aromas if prone to migraines.	Blend rosemary with peppermint for added clarity.

13. Adaptogen Blend for Resilience

Why It Helps

Adaptogens like ashwagandha, rhodiola, and eleuthero rebuild stamina and stress tolerance.

How to Use

- Take 30–40 drops tincture blend twice daily

Quick Remedy	Safety Notes	Variations
Take ashwagandha capsules if short on time.	Avoid rhodiola if very sensitive to stimulation.	Swap rhodiola for holy basil if calming support is preferred.

14. Breath Breaks at the Desk

Why It Helps

Deep breathing calms the nervous system and relieves tension.

How to Use

- Inhale for 5 counts, exhale for 7
- Repeat for 3 minutes, 2–3 times daily

Quick Remedy	Safety Notes	Variations
Even 3 slow breaths between emails resets the body.	Stop if breath-holding feels dizzying.	Pair with aromatherapy using lavender or citrus oils.

15. Lemon Water Reset

Why It Helps

Hydration plus vitamin C refreshes the body and mind, easing fatigue.

How to Use

- Squeeze juice of ½ lemon into 1 cup warm water
- Drink mid-afternoon instead of coffee

Quick Remedy	Safety Notes	Variations
Mix lemon juice into cold water on the go.	Rinse mouth afterward to protect enamel.	Add grated ginger or honey for extra boost.

Case Studies: Two Women's Healing Journeys

Case Study 1: Anna, The Caregiver

Anna was forty-two, caring for her two children and her aging mother. By the time she came to one of my workshops, she was running on four hours of sleep and daily coffee. She felt irritable, tearful, and completely spent. We started small: a nightly oatstraw infusion to calm her nervous system, a lavender foot soak twice a week, and a morning switch from coffee to nettle-peppermint tea.

After a month, she reported, "I still have the same responsibilities, but I no longer feel like I'm drowning. I have small moments of peace in between moments of chaos." Within three months, her cycles stabilized, her sleep improved, and she told me her children said, "You laugh again, Mom."

Case Study 2: Maria, The Professional

Maria was thirty-six, climbing the ladder in a corporate job and also a multi-mile runner. She faced irregular cycles, PMS migraines, and crushing fatigue. She believed she had no time to slow down for "self-care" rituals. We chose simple, targeted remedies: vitex tea each morning, rosemary inhalation before meetings, sage tea for hot flashes that were creeping in during her late-afternoon commutes, and meditation practices.

At first, she worried nothing was changing. By her third cycle, she emailed me: "For the first time in years, I didn't need painkillers on the first day of my period." She now keeps garlic honey at her desk during flu season and makes bone broth once a month on Sundays. "It's not about doing it all," she says. "It's about having allies."

Quick Grab Box: Fastest Women's Remedies

Sometimes you don't have the time or energy for a long ritual. Sometimes you're at work, in the car, or lying awake at midnight when your body suddenly calls for help. That's when the **quick remedies** become your closest allies. They are small, portable, and immediate. Herbs are medicine you can lean on in the busiest corners of your life.

Here are the fastest remedies from this chapter, each one chosen because it can bring relief in minutes:

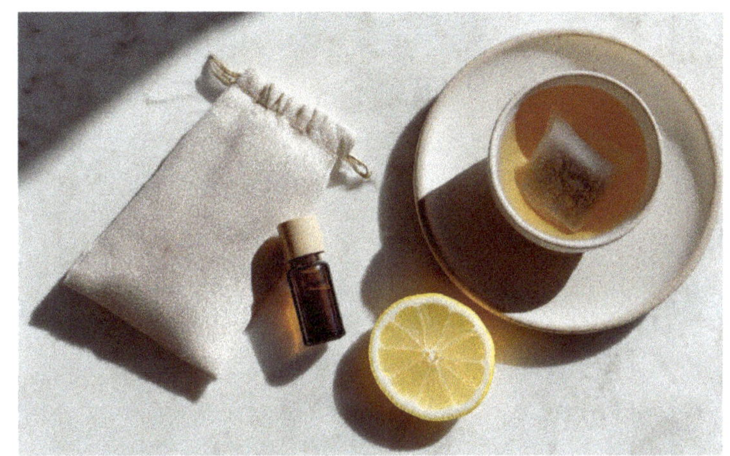

Quick Grab Box: Fastest Women's Remedies

For Menstrual Pain

- **Cramp Bark Tincture (Remedy 2):** 30–40 drops in water. Relief in 20 minutes.

For PMS Mood Swings

- **Lavender Foot Soak (Remedy 10):** ½ cup Epsom salts + 8 drops lavender oil in warm water. Calm within minutes.

For Hot Flashes

- **Sage Tea (Remedy 5):** 1 tsp dried sage in 1 cup hot water. Sip slowly during an episode.

For Energy at Work

- **Rosemary Inhalation (Remedy 12):** Rub a sprig of rosemary between your fingers and inhale deeply.

For Afternoon Fatigue

- **Lemon Water Reset (Remedy 15):** Juice of ½ lemon in warm water. Refreshes body and mind in seconds.

These remedies require no elaborate preparation and can be used at home, in the office, or on the go. They are your portable, practical toolkit for women's wellness.

Why Quick Remedies Build Confidence

The fast-acting remedies are more than emergency helpers. They are confidence builders. When you feel your cramps ease, your mood soften, or your mind sharpen in minutes, you begin to trust your body's response to natural medicine. This trust encourages you to explore the deeper rituals such as overnight infusions, seed cycling, or adaptogen blends without fear or hesitation.

Quick remedies prove that healing is possible now. They give you the courage to stay the course with the longer practices that repair and nourish over time.

Benefit to You

By keeping just a few of these quick remedies at hand, you'll:

- Ease pain or discomfort on the spot.

- Stay grounded during work, family, or emotional demands.

- Prevent overwhelm by knowing you always have a tool ready.

- Strengthen your connection to your body by noticing immediate results.

REMEMBER: you don't need to do everything at once. Choose one quick remedy this week. Carry it in your bag or keep it on your nightstand. Let it prove itself to you. Let it become the beginning of your trust in the gentle, steady power of women's wellness.

Bringing It Together

Women's wellness isn't a luxury. It's a necessity. The remedies in this chapter aren't meant to fix you—because you aren't broken. They're here to steady your cycles, nourish your nerves, and refill the well of energy you give from daily.

When you choose even one ritual—a tea, a soak, a breath, for example—you remind your body that she matters. Healing becomes not something you add on top of an already full life but something woven into the life you are already living.

Action Steps

- Choose one remedy from the hormonal harmony section that speaks to your current need (vitex for cycles, sage for hot flashes, cramp bark for pain).

- Add one cycle/nervous system nourishment (raspberry leaf tea, oatstraw infusion, magnesium snack).

- Adopt one energy ritual that you can practice at work or home (rosemary inhalation, lemon water, breath breaks).

- Reflect at the end of the month: Which remedies felt most supportive? Which would you like to carry forward long term?

Bonus Content

Pause and reflect. Scan the QR to download the **Self-Healing Reflection Journal Pages**, printable templates for daily check-ins, weekly wins, and nervous-system resets as you build new habits.

CHAPTER SEVEN

Healing for Busy Bodies and Burnt-Out Minds

> "Until man duplicates a blade of grass, nature can laugh at his so-called scientific knowledge. Remedies from chemicals will never stand in favor compared with the products of nature, the living cell of the plant, the final result of the rays of the sun, the mother of all life."
>
> — *Thomas A. Edison*

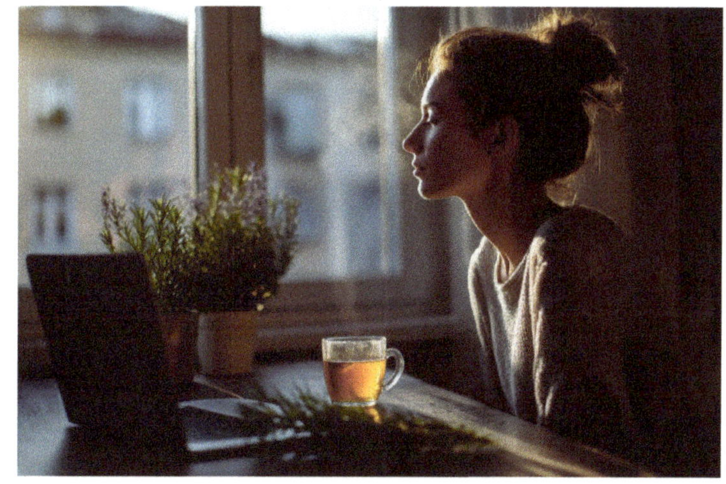

I see it everywhere: the hunched shoulders at the grocery checkout, the quick inhale before answering a question, the tired eyes staring into a glowing screen at 10 p.m. Our modern world asks us to go faster than the human body was designed to. The result is exhaustion—burnt-out minds, tired bodies, frayed nerves.

I know this not just from teaching but from my own seasons of burnout. When I was raising two children while teaching workshops and tending the garden, I used to believe I could power through. I drank too much coffee, skipped meals, answered emails at midnight, and wore my fatigue like a badge of honor. Look how much I could get done in one day—I thought I was fantastic.

However, my body thought otherwise and finally said no: constant colds, migraines, and a deep sadness that I couldn't shake.

What saved me weren't complicated regimens, it was actually small and repeatable resets. A morning tonic that woke me gently instead of jolting me. A rosemary sprig I kept in my pocket to sniff before walking into stressful meetings. A nightly ritual of magnesium baths. None of these took more than a few minutes, but they created space for my nervous system to recover.

This chapter is written for anyone who says: *"I don't have time for healing."* Well, you do if you care to make the time. In fact, the busier you are, the more you need these quick anchors.

Here, you will find remedies that take 5–10 minutes at most, along with a nervous system reset checklist and a quick grab box you can carry with you anywhere. These practices won't just reduce symptoms in the moment. They will remind you that relief is possible, even in the busiest life!

Reset Routines (Remedies 1–4)

1. Morning Reset: Lemon-Ginger Wake-Up

Why It Helps

Instead of jolting the system with coffee, lemon and ginger stimulate digestion, circulation, and focus gently.

How to Use

- Juice of ½ lemon
- 2 slices fresh ginger
- 1 cup warm water

    Steep 5 minutes. Drink first thing in the morning.

Quick Remedy	Safety Notes	Variations
Simply squeeze lemon into warm water if ginger isn't on hand.	Use caution with ginger if prone to acid reflux.	Add a pinch of turmeric for anti-inflammatory support.

2. Morning Reset: Breath & Stretch Ritual

Why It Helps

Five minutes of movement and breath shifts the nervous system from sleep to wakefulness without shock.

How to Use

- Stand tall, feet grounded
- Inhale, arms overhead, stretch long; exhale, arms wide

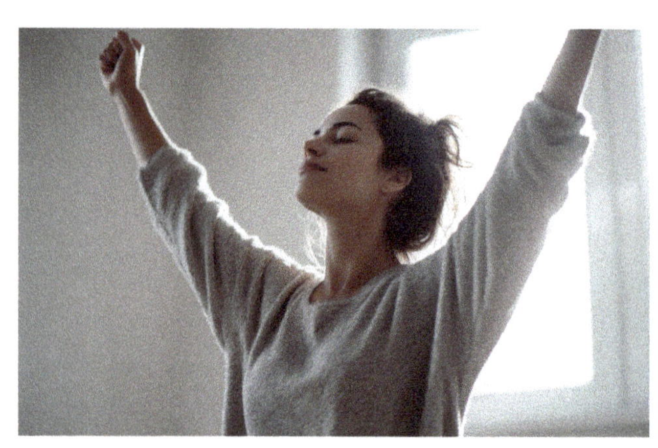

- Repeat 5 times

- Practice 5 cycles of 4-7-8 breathing (inhale 4, hold 7, exhale 8)

Quick Remedy	Safety Notes	Variations
Do while the kettle boils.	If holding breath feels uncomfortable, shorten counts but keep ratio.	Pair with diffused citrus oil for added brightness.

3. Workday Reset: Rosemary Clarity Jar

Why It Helps

Rosemary stimulates blood flow to the brain and improves focus.

How to Use

- Fill a small jar with dried rosemary

- Open and inhale deeply for 30 seconds when brain fog hits

Quick Remedy	Safety Notes	Variations
Rub fresh rosemary between fingers and sniff.	Avoid strong aromas if prone to migraines.	Blend dried peppermint into the jar for a sharper lift.

4. Evening Reset: Magnesium-Lavender Bath

Why It Helps

Transdermal magnesium relaxes muscles; lavender oil calms the nervous system.

How to Use

- 1 cup Epsom salts

- 10 drops lavender essential oil

  Add to a warm bath and soak 20 minutes before bed.

Quick Remedy	Safety Notes	Variations
Use a 10-minute foot soak if no tub.	Avoid very hot baths if you have high blood pressure.	Add rose petals or chamomile to bathwater for comfort.

Five-Minute Fixes (Remedies 5–8)

5. Anxiety Ease: Chamomile Hand Compress

Why It Helps

Chamomile relaxes both muscles and the mind through warmth and aroma.

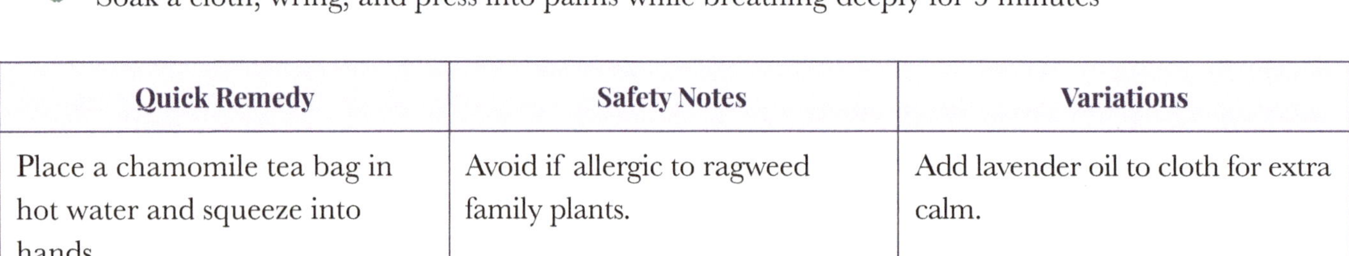

How to Use

- Brew 2 tbsp dried chamomile in 2 cups hot water for 10 minutes
- Soak a cloth, wring, and press into palms while breathing deeply for 3 minutes

Quick Remedy	Safety Notes	Variations
Place a chamomile tea bag in hot water and squeeze into hands.	Avoid if allergic to ragweed family plants.	Add lavender oil to cloth for extra calm.

6. Tension Release: Shoulder Oil Massage

Why It Helps

Self-massage with warming oils relieves tension in shoulders and neck.

How to Use

- Dilute 2 drops rosemary essential oil in 1 tsp olive oil
- Massage into shoulders, neck, and temples for 3 minutes

Quick Remedy	Safety Notes	Variations
Keep a pre-made roll-on with rosemary oil in your bag.	Avoid near eyes. Test oil dilution on skin first.	Blend with lavender oil for a relaxing version.

7. Brain Fog Fix: Peppermint Steam

Why It Helps

Peppermint clears sinuses and stimulates alertness.

How to Use

- 1 tsp dried peppermint
- 1 cup boiling water

Pour into a bowl, lean over, cover head with towel, inhale 3 minutes.

Quick Remedy	Safety Notes	Variations
Sip peppermint tea if steam isn't possible.	Avoid steam burns—keep face at safe distance.	Add eucalyptus leaves for stronger vapors.

8. Mood Lift: Citrus Inhale

Why It Helps

Citrus oils like sweet orange trigger serotonin release and ease tension.

How to Use

- Place 1 drop orange essential oil on a cotton ball
- Inhale deeply for 1 minute

Quick Remedy	Safety Notes	Variations
Carry in a small baggie and reuse.	Avoid applying citrus oils directly to skin before sun exposure.	Blend orange and bergamot oils for deeper uplift.

Wind-Down Rituals (Remedies 9–11)

9. Digital Sunset: Blue Light Break

Why It Helps

Blue light disrupts melatonin, making sleep harder. Turning screens off resets circadian rhythm.

How to Use

- Shut down devices 30 minutes before bed
- Replace scrolling with tea, journaling, or stretching

Quick Remedy	Safety Notes	Variations
Use blue-light blocking glasses if device use is unavoidable.	Ensure glasses block 90%+ of blue light for best effect.	Create a bedroom ritual with candlelight instead of screens.

10. Hops & Chamomile Sleep Sachet

Why It Helps

Hops are mildly sedative, and chamomile soothes the nervous system, together they gently encourage sleep.

How to Use

- 2 tbsp dried hops + 1 tbsp dried chamomile
- Fill a small breathable sachet, squeeze before bed, tuck by pillow
- Replace every 4–6 weeks or when scent fades

Quick Remedy	Safety Notes	Variations
Tuck a cooled chamomile tea bag in your pillowcase.	Avoid if pregnant, breastfeeding, or taking sedatives; keep out of reach of infants; don't apply essential oils directly to children's skin.	Swap hops for 1–2 tsp dried lemon balm for a milder, lemony calming sachet

11. Gratitude Journaling

Why It Helps

Noting small gratitudes rewires the brain toward calm and contentment.

How to Use

- Each night, write down 3 things you're grateful for
- Keep notebook by bed for consistency

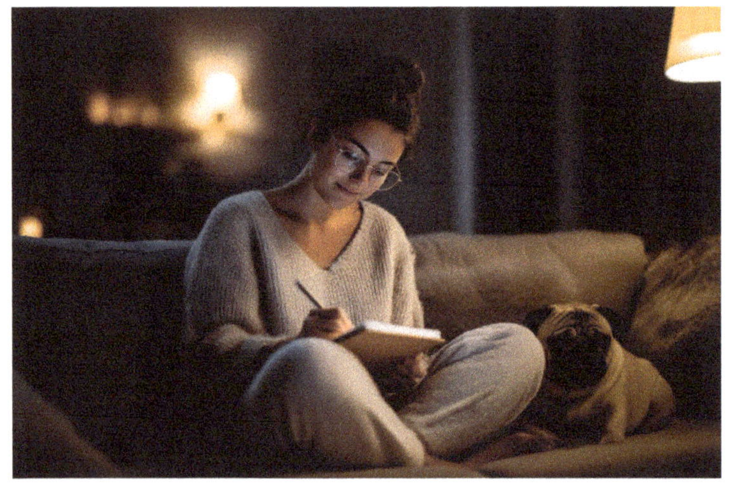

Quick Remedy	Safety Notes	Variations
Say gratitudes aloud if you can't write.	None needed—safe and beneficial for all.	Add a calming tea ritual before journaling.

Nervous System Reset Checklist

1. **Pause for Breath:** Practice 4-7-8 breathing for 3 rounds.
2. **Sip Something Warm:** Chamomile, lemon balm, or hot water with lemon.
3. **Inhale an Aroma:** Rosemary for clarity, lavender for calm, citrus for uplift.

4. **Touch Ritual:** Warm compress on hands or shoulders.
5. **Write One Line:** Note what you feel; naming reduces overwhelm.

This sequence takes under 10 minutes. Use in the car before heading home, during lunch, or right before bed.

Quick Grab Box: 3 Remedies to Keep in Your Bag

* **Lavender Oil Roller:** Swipe on wrists when anxiety spikes.
* **Rosemary Sprig or Dried Jar:** Inhale when brain fog rolls in.
* **Orange Oil Cotton Ball:** Quick mood lift for fatigue or low days.

Together, these three weigh less than a lipstick tube, yet they cover the most common struggles of daily stress.

Bringing It Together

Burnout doesn't just vanish overnight. However, it can soften when you build small islands of rest into your day. These eleven remedies aren't about changing your whole life, they're about reclaiming a few minutes here and there. The nervous system is remarkably responsive. A single breath, a single aroma, a single soak can begin to rewire how your body carries stress.

Healing isn't something you "add" to your schedule. It's something you weave into what you already do. It also takes time and patience to heal from the root, which is what herbalism is all about. Lemon water instead of your second coffee. Rosemary sniff instead of a third scroll through your phone. Lavender bath instead of collapsing into bed with tension still in your shoulders.

Start with one remedy. Let it remind you that you are not powerless. Relief is closer than you think!

Bonus Content

You're ready to make a plan. Scan the QR to download the **Beginner's Remedy Planner**, a simple worksheet to choose 3–5 remedies, schedule them, and track your progress.

CHAPTER EIGHT

Healing in the City

> "Even a wounded world is feeding us. Even a wounded world holds us, giving us moments of wonder and joy. I choose joy over despair. Not because I have my head in the sand but because joy is what the earth gives me daily and I must return the gift."
>
> — *Robin Wall Kimmerer*

I have met many people who believe herbal healing is only possible if you have a garden in the backyard, a shed filled with jars, and endless time to prepare remedies. It is a beautiful dream, but the truth is: Most of us live in cities, or at least in apartments with limited space and little spare time. Life in the city can feel like the opposite of natural wellness, with its artificial bright lights, crowded commutes, fast food, long hours indoors, and loud noises. I hear the same refrain often: "I'd love to use herbs, but it doesn't fit my life."

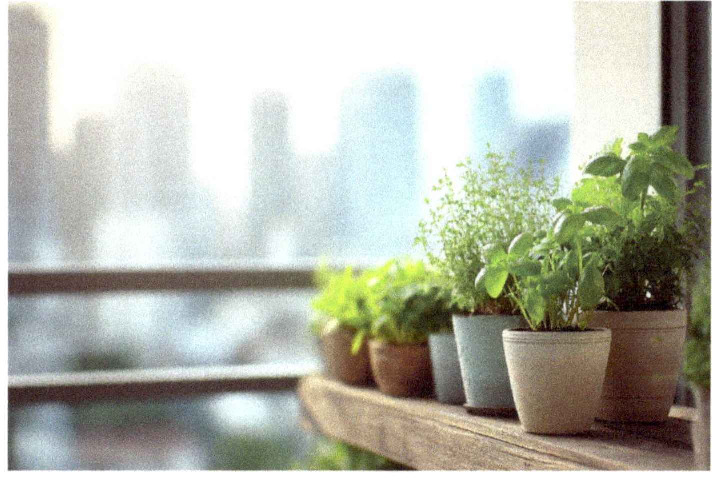

The truth is that healing belongs to everyone. You don't need acres of land or a country kitchen to care for yourself naturally—although that would be amazing. Herbs and rituals adapt beautifully to urban life. A tea bag tucked in your desk drawer, a tincture bottle in your handbag, or a few pots of basil and mint on the windowsill… these are just as valid as a meadow full of wildflowers.

When I first moved to Oregon, I met a young woman at one of my workshops who lived on the 14th floor of a downtown apartment. She told me she felt cut off from nature and thought she couldn't practice herbalism until she moved somewhere "greener." I asked her to show me what she carried in her purse that day. She pulled out a packet of chamomile tea, a small lavender lip balm, and a bottle of water. I smiled and said, "You already have your apothecary right here." Her eyes lit up. She had been practicing healing all along, just without realizing it.

This chapter is for the city dwellers, the apartment renters, the busy professionals who long for wellness but feel blocked by space, time, or access. Here, you'll learn:

- The best herbs to buy pre-made so you don't have to DIY everything.

- Simple grounding rituals you can do even in the middle of a concrete jungle.

- A few "healing-in-your-handbag" allies that travel with you wherever you go.

Healing doesn't have to wait until you move to the countryside or retire into free time. It can live in your studio apartment, your subway commute, your work bag. The earth meets us where we are, and yes, even between tall buildings and neon lights!

The Best Herbs to Buy Pre-Made

One of the biggest barriers I hear from city dwellers is time. "I don't have hours to simmer syrups or space to dry herbs," they say. And they're right! Life in the city moves quickly and can be overstimulating. That doesn't mean you can't use herbs—it actually means you probably really need their support, particularly for your nervous and immune systems. It also means you need allies that are easy, reliable, and ready when you are.

Buying pre-made doesn't make your practice less "authentic," either! In fact, it can be wise. Herbalists throughout history have traded, purchased, and shared remedies. My grandmother made her own tinctures, but she also bought teas at the co-op and kept pre-packaged calendula salve in her bathroom cabinet. The truth is: what matters most is actually using the remedy, not how much time you spent making it.

Here are a few of the best herbal allies to buy pre-made when you live in the city:

Section 1: Best Herbs to Buy Pre-Made

Chamomile Tea Bags

Why It Helps

Chamomile eases digestion, reduces anxiety, and supports sleep. Studies show chamomile extract can significantly improve sleep quality in those with insomnia.

How to Use

- 1 tea bag chamomile

- 1 cup hot water

  Steep 10 minutes, covered. Drink after meals or before bed.

Quick Remedy	Safety Notes	Variations
Carry a few tea bags in your wallet or bag—any café or office can provide hot water.	Avoid if allergic to ragweed family plants.	Add honey or lemon for flavor.

Peppermint Tea Bags

Why It Helps

Peppermint sharpens focus, eases bloating, and clears brain fog. In one small study, peppermint improved alertness during demanding mental tasks.

How to Use

* 1 tsp dried peppermint or 1 tea bag
* 1 cup hot water

   Steep 5 minutes. Drink in afternoon slump.

Quick Remedy	Safety Notes	Variations
Rub a sprig of fresh mint between your fingers and inhale.	Avoid strong peppermint tea if prone to reflux.	Blend with chamomile for both calm and clarity.

Elderberry Syrup (Pre-Made)

Why It Helps

Elderberries are rich in flavonoids that strengthen immunity. Studies show elderberry syrup can shorten colds if taken early.

How to Use

* 1 tsp daily for prevention
* 1 tbsp every few hours at first sign of illness

Quick Remedy	Safety Notes	Variations
Keep a travel-sized bottle in your fridge or desk.	Don't consume raw elderberries; syrup is safe once cooked.	Choose blends with ginger or cinnamon for extra warmth.

Ready-Made Tinctures

Why It Helps

Tinctures are concentrated, shelf-stable extracts. Lemon balm for anxiety, valerian for sleep, echinacea for immunity—each works quickly.

How to Use

* Take 30–40 drops in a splash of water as needed

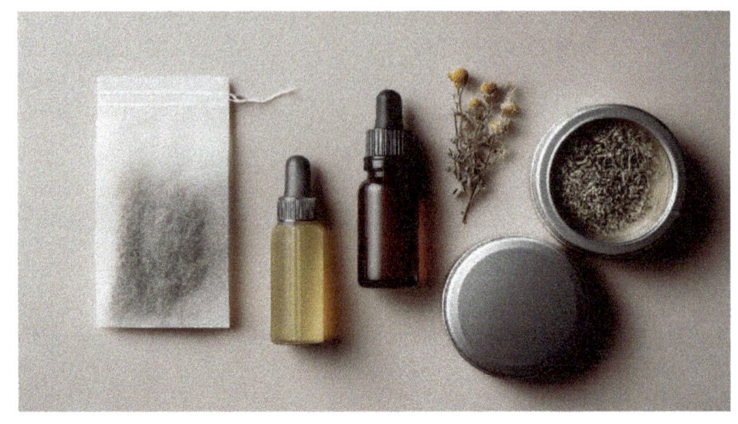

Quick Remedy	Safety Notes	Variations
Carry a 1-oz dropper bottle in your bag—relief in under 20 minutes.	Check labels for alcohol content if avoiding.	Blend lemon balm and skullcap for calm focus.

Salves and Balms

Why It Helps

Calendula or arnica salves soothe dry skin, bruises, or sore muscles.

How to Use

* Apply pea-sized amount to affected area

Quick Remedy	Safety Notes	Variations
Slip a travel tin into your bag for emergencies.	Avoid open wounds unless salve is specifically for cuts.	Lavender balm doubles as both skin care and aromatherapy.

Section 2: Urban Grounding Rituals

Morning Coffee Alternative: Lemon Water Reset

Why It Helps

Lemon water hydrates and gently stimulates digestion.

How to Use

* Juice of ½ lemon
* 1 cup warm water
  Sip slowly in the morning.

Quick Remedy	Safety Notes	Variations
Carry a small lemon in your bag and ask for hot water at cafés.	Rinse mouth after to protect enamel.	Add grated ginger for extra warmth.

Midday Pause: Pocket Breathing

Why It Helps

Breath is the fastest way to calm the nervous system. Slow exhalation lowers heart rate.

How to Use

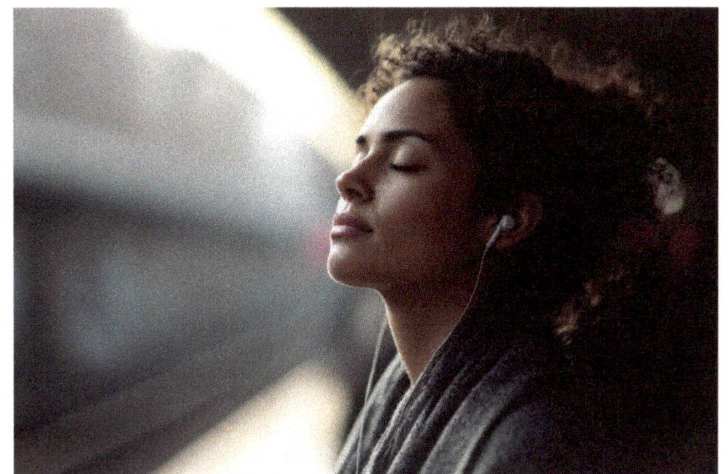

- Inhale through nose for 4 counts
- Exhale through mouth for 6 counts

  Repeat 5 rounds at your desk or on the subway.

Quick Remedy	Safety Notes	Variations
Do three slow breaths while waiting for an elevator.	None—safe and beneficial for all.	Pair with lavender oil on wrists.

Evening Ritual: Rooftop or Balcony Herbs

Why It Helps

Even small pots of basil, mint, or thyme reconnect city dwellers to living plants. Touching and smelling them lowers stress.

How to Use

- Keep 2–3 small herb pots on a windowsill or balcony
- Snip leaves for tea or meals

Quick Remedy	Safety Notes	Variations
Even rubbing leaves between fingers for scent is grounding.	Ensure herbs receive 4–6 hours sunlight.	Try microgreens indoors with grow lights.

Section 3: Healing in Your Handbag

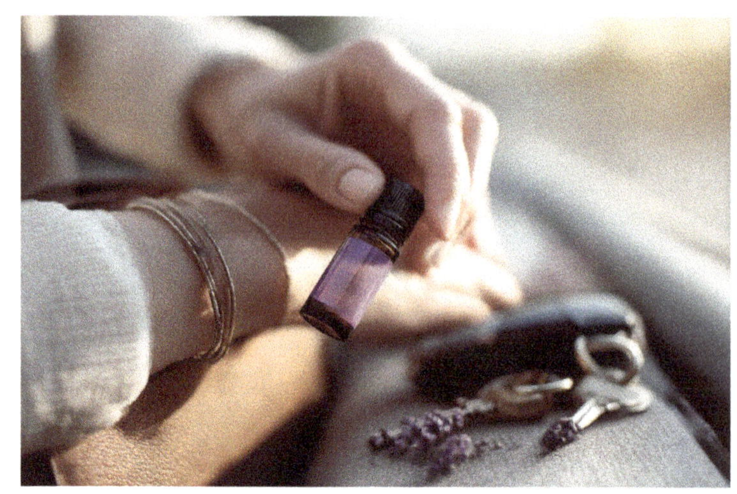

Lavender Roller Bottle

Why It Helps

Lavender oil calms anxiety and lowers stress hormones.

How to Use

* Dilute 10 drops lavender oil in 2 tbsp carrier oil
* Apply to wrists, temples, or neck as needed

Quick Remedy	Safety Notes	Variations
Swipe and inhale before stressful meetings or commutes.	Avoid eyes. Test on small patch first.	Blend lavender with bergamot for uplift.

Elderberry Lozenges

Why It Helps

Soothe a scratchy throat while delivering immune support.

How to Use

* Dissolve one lozenge slowly in mouth as needed

Quick Remedy	Safety Notes	Variations
Carry in bag during cold season or on airplanes.	Choose sugar-free if monitoring blood sugar.	Opt for blends with zinc or vitamin C.

Chamomile Tea Stash

Why It Helps

A single tea bag can turn any stressful office into a calm moment.

How to Use

* Steep in hot water 10 minutes during tension

Quick Remedy	Safety Notes	Variations
Simply inhale the warm steam while steeping.	Avoid if allergic to ragweed.	Pair with peppermint for stress + focus.

Section 4: Five-Minute Fixes for City Stress

Hand Compress for Tension

Why It Helps

Warmth plus herbs relax tight muscles quickly.

How to Use

- Brew 2 chamomile or lavender tea bags in 2 cups hot water

- Soak washcloth, wring, and press into hands for 5 minutes

Quick Remedy	Safety Notes	Variations
Microwave damp cloth with 2 drops lavender oil.	Avoid burns—let cloth cool to comfortable warmth.	Use peppermint for refreshing lift.

Rosemary "Subway Sniff"

Why It Helps

Rosemary increases alertness and sharpens memory.

How to Use

- Keep dried rosemary in a small jar

- Inhale deeply for 30 seconds during commute

Quick Remedy	Safety Notes	Variations
Rub a sprig between fingers and sniff.	Avoid if strong scents trigger headaches.	Blend rosemary with peppermint leaves.

Citrus Cotton Ball

Why It Helps

Citrus aroma uplifts mood and reduces anxiety.

How to Use

- Place 1 drop orange or lemon oil on cotton ball
- Inhale for 1–2 minutes during stressful moments

Quick Remedy	Safety Notes	Variations
Keep in a resealable baggie to reuse.	Avoid direct skin contact followed by sun exposure.	Use bergamot for deeper calm.

Section 5: Morning-to-Evening Reset Ideas

Morning: Start with lemon water reset instead of coffee. Take vitex tea or maca powder if supporting hormones. Carry chamomile or peppermint tea bags for the day.

Midday: Use rosemary sniff jar or citrus cotton ball during work breaks. Add fermented foods like sauerkraut to your lunch for digestive and immune support.

Afternoon: Drink nettle-peppermint tea instead of an energy drink. Keep elderberry lozenges at your desk during cold season.

Evening: Shut down screens thirty minutes before bed. Brew chamomile tea, soak feet with lavender salts, or keep a lavender pillow sachet by your bed.

Even in a busy city schedule, these micro-rituals weave healing into what you're already doing.

Quick Grab Box: Fastest Urban Remedies

- **Chamomile Tea Bag:** Stress, digestion, sleep—portable and easy.
- **Rosemary Sniff Jar:** Brain fog fix during commutes or late workdays.
- **Lavender Roller Bottle:** Calm anxiety in seconds.
- **Elderberry Lozenge:** Daily immune support in crowded spaces.

These four remedies fit into a small handbag yet cover most of what urban life demands: stress relief, focus, calm, and immunity.

Closing Reflection

Healing doesn't wait for perfect conditions. It doesn't require acreage, silence, or endless time. It happens in kitchens the size of closets, on noisy subways, under fluorescent lights. Herbs meet us where we are.

A tea bag in your desk drawer. A roller bottle in your bag. A pot of mint on your balcony. These are small acts, but they carry the same wisdom as the wild meadow. They remind us: *I am connected. I am cared for. I am capable of tending myself, even here.*

Start with one. Carry chamomile tomorrow. Inhale rosemary before your next meeting. Let lavender meet you at bedtime. These small choices ripple out, softening the edges of city life, guiding you back to balance—one sip, one breath, one pocket-sized ally at a time.

CHAPTER NINE

Building Healing Habits That Stick

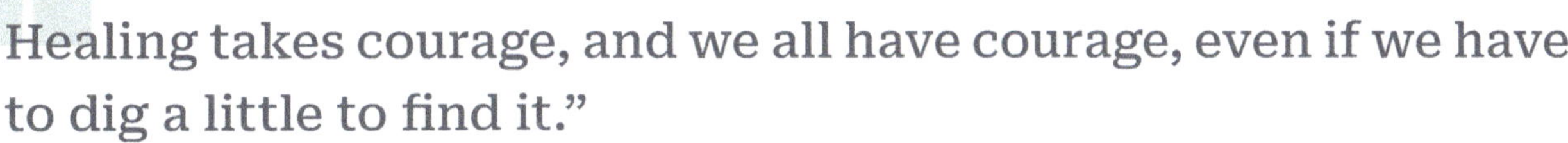

"Healing takes courage, and we all have courage, even if we have to dig a little to find it."

— *Tori Amos*

When I look back at my own healing journey, the biggest shifts never came from one dramatic remedy. They came from the little things I did again and again. Stirring oatstraw infusion each evening before bed. Taking a walk after dinner instead of rushing to my desk. Choosing tea instead of a second coffee. These choices seemed so small, but over weeks, they built resilience.

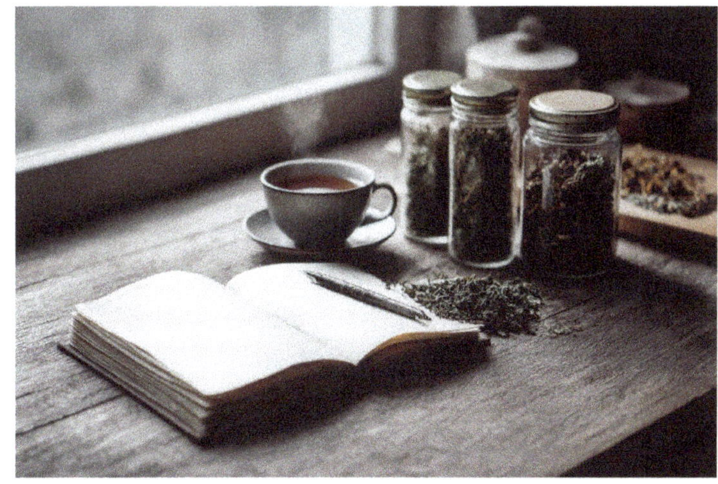

This chapter isn't about learning new remedies—it's about weaving the remedies you already know into your life in ways that last. Many people try herbs with excitement, only to give up after a week because they "forget." The truth is: Our culture doesn't teach us how to build habits that nourish.

Herbs become most powerful when they're part of a rhythm, not a one-time experiment.

Here, you'll discover gentle routines for energy, digestion, and focus, ideas for monthly and seasonal check-ins, and journal prompts that help you notice your wins along the way. These practices are how you turn a chapter of a book into a living, breathing lifestyle.

Gentle Routines for Energy, Digestion, and Focus

Morning Energy: Nettle–Peppermint Start

Why It Helps

Nettle replenishes minerals, while peppermint clears morning fog. This ritual replaces overstimulation with steady energy.

How to Use

- 1 tbsp dried nettle
- 1 tsp dried peppermint
- 2 cups hot water

    Steep 15 minutes. Drink in the morning as you begin your day.

Quick Remedy	Safety Notes	Variations
Steep 1 tsp each in a travel mug for 5 minutes if rushed.	Mildly diuretic—drink water alongside.	Add lemon for brightness.

Midday Digestion: Bitters Before Lunch

Why It Helps

Bitters stimulate digestive juices, improving nutrient absorption and preventing sluggishness.

How to Use

- Take 20–30 drops of dandelion or gentian tincture in water 10 minutes before meals.

Quick Remedy	Safety Notes	Variations
If tincture isn't on hand, chew a small handful of arugula or radicchio before eating.	Avoid gentian if you have ulcers or very sensitive stomach.	Try orange peel or chamomile bitters for a gentler effect.

Afternoon Focus: Rosemary Sniff Break

Why It Helps

Rosemary has been shown to improve memory and concentration by increasing cerebral blood flow.

How to Use

- Inhale deeply from a jar of dried rosemary or rub a sprig between your fingers.

Quick Remedy	Safety Notes	Variations
Keep a cotton ball with a drop of rosemary oil in a baggie.	Avoid strong scents if prone to headaches.	Blend rosemary with peppermint for extra lift.

Evening Wind-Down: Chamomile or Lemon Balm Tea

Why It Helps

Both herbs ease the nervous system, improve digestion, and prepare the body for rest.

How to Use

- 1 tsp dried chamomile or lemon balm
- 1 cup hot water

    Steep 10 minutes. Drink after dinner or before bed.

Quick Remedy	Safety Notes	Variations
Use tea bags when traveling or exhausted.	Avoid lemon balm in large doses with hypothyroidism.	Add rose petals for heart-soothing calm.

Monthly Check-Ins and Seasonal Rhythms

Monthly Self-Check

Why It Helps

Healing becomes more sustainable when you pause regularly to notice patterns.

How to Use

At the end of each month, write down:
- What remedies you used most
- How your energy, digestion, mood, or sleep shifted
- What felt easy, what felt hard

Quick Remedy	Safety Notes	Variations
Set a calendar reminder for the last Sunday of each month.	None—safe and reflective practice.	Share reflections with a friend or support group.

Seasonal Shifts

Why It Helps

Aligning habits with seasons honors both body and nature. In Traditional Chinese Medicine and Western herbalism alike, the seasons guide how we eat, rest, and prepare.

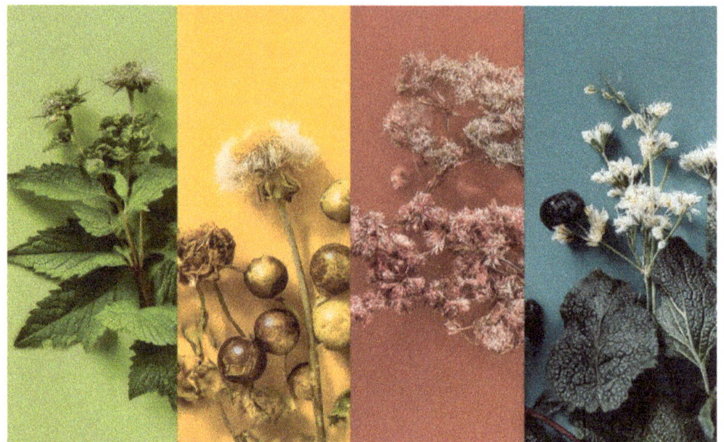

How to Use

- **Spring:** Focus on cleansing greens like dandelion, nettle, arugula
- **Summer:** Hydrating herbs like hibiscus, mint, lemon balm
- **Autumn:** Immune builders like elderberry, astragalus, garlic
- **Winter:** Restoratives like ashwagandha, oatstraw, chamomile

Quick Remedy	Safety Notes	Variations
Add one seasonal herb to your daily tea.	Introduce new herbs slowly to monitor reactions.	Journal what seasonal herbs make you feel most supported.

Self-Reflection Prompts: "Healing Wins & Lessons"

Reflection keeps healing alive. Too often, we dismiss our progress because we expect dramatic results. By recording even small changes, you build momentum and self-trust.

Prompts to Use Monthly:

- *This month, I felt proud when I…*
- *A small win I noticed in my energy or mood was…*
- *One lesson I learned about my body was…*
- *A ritual that felt easy and joyful was…*
- *A place I'd like to give myself more support is…*

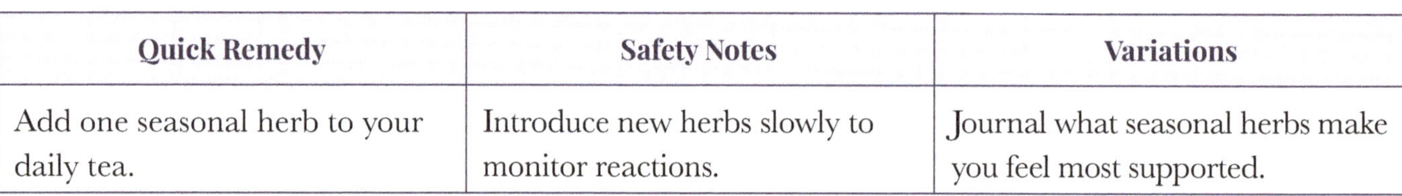

Quick Remedy
Jot down one "healing win" on a sticky note each week. Collect them in a jar to read at year's end.

Habit Anchors: Turning Rituals into Rhythms

When I first began drinking nettle infusion, I thought the challenge would be making it. It turned out the real challenge was remembering to make it. I would buy my herbs, put them in glass jars, and tell myself, *"I'll start tomorrow."* Then tomorrow became next week. I simply didn't yet have a rhythm.

That's when I learned about habit anchors. Instead of relying on willpower, I paired each herbal ritual with something I was already doing. I made nettle tea while waiting for my morning coffee to brew. I lit a candle for my evening lemon balm tea as I brushed my teeth. I tucked lavender oil into my bag next to my keys so I'd see it every time I left the house.

Anchors are how small acts become automatic. Over time, the nettle wasn't a "new habit" anymore, it was simply part of how I started my day.

How to Use

- Pick one herbal ritual you want to keep (like evening chamomile tea).

- Attach it to something you already do daily (like brushing teeth or washing dishes).

- Repeat consistently until the two are linked in your mind.

Quick Remedy	Safety Notes
Choose one anchor today. Place a jar, tea bag, or tincture right next to an item you already use (like your coffee pot or toothbrush).	Experiment with morning, midday, and evening anchors to see which flow most easily.

Seasonal Journal Rituals

Herbs teach us to pay attention to cycles. Plants change with the seasons, and so do we. Too often in city or office life, seasons blur into each other—we live by clocks and screens instead of natural rhythms. By keeping a seasonal journal, you give yourself a way to track not just remedies but also your body's relationship to time.

Each season, I sit with a cup of tea and ask myself: *What do I need now?* In spring, my answer is often greens and movement. In summer, it is hydration and cooling herbs. In autumn, warmth and immune support. In winter, more rest. My body rarely lies—it just needs me to listen.

How to Use

At the start of each season, ask:

- What herbs am I drawn to?

- How is my body asking me to slow down or speed up?

- What one small habit can I keep this season?

Write reflections in a dedicated notebook.

Quick Remedy	Safety Notes
If you're short on time, jot one line in your phone notes app each equinox and solstice.	Pair your seasonal journal ritual with a walk outdoors, even in the city—notice what's blooming, fading, or resting.

Healing in Community

Another reason habits fail is that we try to do everything alone. Healing is deeply personal, yes—but it is also communal. For centuries, women gathered in kitchens, markets, and fields to share remedies. They reminded each other to take their teas, swapped tinctures, and encouraged rest.

I've seen the difference it makes when people gather, even virtually. One of my students, Sarah, began a "Tea Tuesday" group chat with three friends. Every Tuesday at 8 p.m., they all made tea—sometimes chamomile, sometimes nettle—and texted each other a photo of their mug. Within weeks, tea had gone from "optional" to non-negotiable. The accountability wasn't harsh—it was joyful.

How to Use

* Invite one friend or family member to share a ritual with you.

* Choose a time—weekly or monthly—when you'll check in with each other.

* Share not just what you drank but how it made you feel.

Quick Remedy	Safety Notes
If you can't gather in person, send a simple text: *"Tea time?"*	Expand into seasonal potlucks, where each person brings a dish or drink featuring a healing herb.

Reflection: The Power of Small Wins

We underestimate the power of noticing progress. A client once told me she had "failed" at her oatstraw habit because she only managed to brew it twice in a month. I asked her: *"Before this, how often did you drink oatstraw?"* She laughed: *"Never."*

Twice is not failure—it is progress. The key is to name those wins. Your nervous system thrives on encouragement. Each time you acknowledge that you *did* show up, you create momentum.

How to Use

* End each week by writing one line: *"One healing act I did this week was…"*

* Collect these notes in a jar, notebook, or calendar.

Quick Remedy	Safety Notes
If writing feels like too much, speak your win aloud before bed.	Turn it into a family ritual—invite children or partners to share their own healing wins.

Bringing It Together

Habits are what carry herbs from occasional experiments into lifelong allies. Your body thrives on rhythm. By pairing simple remedies with daily moments—morning nettle, midday bitters, afternoon rosemary, evening chamomile—you create a framework of support.

The monthly check-ins and seasonal shifts remind you that healing isn't static. It flows with your life. Some months you'll be consistent, others you'll forget. Both are fine. What matters is returning, gently, without shame.

Begin with one daily anchor and one monthly reflection. That's enough. Over time, your remedies will become second nature—woven into meals, commutes, bedtime. This is how herbs move from your shelf into your life.

When you turn the page, we'll explore how to keep expanding your healing journey with community, connection, and deeper practices that sustain not only your health but your sense of belonging.

Bonus Content

Ready to make these habits real? Scan the QR to download the **30-Day Natural Healing Challenge** (printable PDF) and start today.

CHAPTER TEN

Earth Medicine for the Family

> " The way you help heal the world is you start with your own family."

> — *Mother Teresa*

Healing is never just personal. From the moment we brew tea for a child, rub balm on a partner's sore shoulders, or stir honey into warm water for a friend, healing expands into the fabric of family. Herbs are not solitary—they are communal, passed from one generation to the next, shared at kitchen tables, offered in moments of need.

I still remember when my daughter came home from school with her first cold. She was five years old, her nose red, her eyes watery, her body limp. Instead of rushing for medicine, I wrapped her in a blanket, brewed chamomile tea, and stirred in honey. She sipped slowly, her breathing eased, and she fell asleep in my lap. That moment taught me: Earth medicine isn't just about remedies—it's about presence.

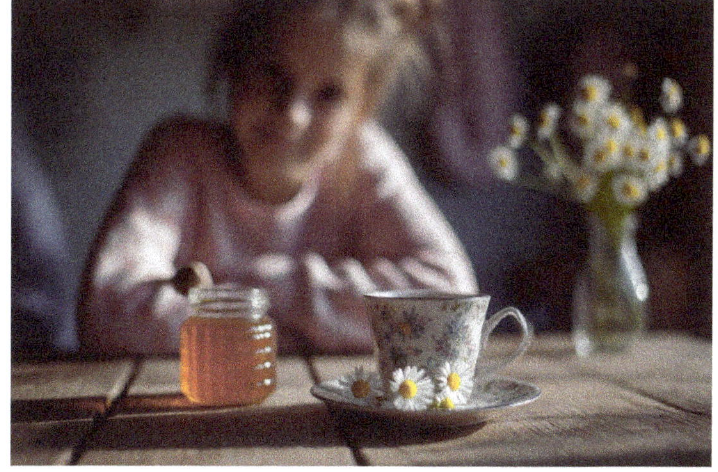

In this chapter, we'll explore practical, family-friendly remedies: gentle teas for children, soothing rubs for partners, safe herbs for pets, and simple kitchen cures for everyday complaints. Each is designed to empower you to offer natural care confidently, knowing you're helping those you love with safe, approachable allies.

Kid-Safe Remedies

Children respond beautifully to herbs when they are used gently and thoughtfully. Their systems are smaller and more sensitive, which means they need much lighter doses than adults, but it also means the effects can be surprisingly profound. When I first began practicing, I was amazed at how quickly chamomile soothed a child's colic, or how a simple oat bath quieted the itch of chickenpox. These are the remedies that often become family traditions—passed down from grandmothers, scribbled on recipe cards, whispered between mothers at playgrounds.

1. Chamomile Honey Tea for Tummy Upsets

Why It Helps

Chamomile calms digestion and relaxes muscle spasms. Honey soothes irritation. Studies show chamomile extract can reduce colic in infants when used appropriately.

How to Use

- 1 tsp dried chamomile or 1 tea bag
- 1 cup hot water Steep 5–7 minutes, strain well

  For children 2+: Add 1 tsp honey and let cool before serving

Quick Remedy	Safety Notes	Variations
Offer a few warm sips during mild nausea or upset stomach.	Avoid honey for children under 1 year. Avoid chamomile if allergic to ragweed family plants.	Add a small slice of fresh ginger for older kids.

2. Oat Bath for Skin Irritation

Why It Helps

Oats are rich in beta-glucans, compounds that soothe itchy, irritated skin from rashes or eczema.

How to Use

- Blend 1 cup oats into fine powder
- Add to warm bathwater
- Let child soak 15 minutes

Quick Remedy	Safety Notes	Variations
Tie oats in a muslin bag and swish through bathwater.	Avoid very hot baths for children.	Add a few drops lavender oil for calming effect (only for children over 3).

3. Elderberry Syrup for Immune Support

Why It Helps

Elderberries strengthen the immune system and reduce severity of colds.

How to Use

- ½ cup dried elderberries
- 3 cups water
- 1 cinnamon stick, 2 cloves, 1 inch ginger Simmer 30 minutes, strain, and stir in 1 cup honey once cooled.
- Give children 1 tsp daily for prevention or 1 tsp every 2–3 hours when sick.

Quick Remedy	Safety Notes	Variations
Use pre-made child-friendly elderberry syrup.	Avoid raw elderberries—they are toxic. Honey only for children over 1.	Swap honey for maple syrup for children under 2.

Partner-Friendly Remedies

4. Arnica Salve for Sore Muscles

Why It Helps

Arnica reduces inflammation and speeds healing after strain.

How to Use

- Apply pea-sized amount to sore areas 2–3 times daily

Quick Remedy	Safety Notes	Variations
Massage gently into shoulders or lower back after long days.	Do not use on broken skin.	Combine with peppermint oil for cooling relief.

5. Ashwagandha Night Tonic for Stress

Why It Helps

Ashwagandha reduces cortisol and supports better sleep, easing tension after work.

How to Use

- 1 tsp ashwagandha powder
- 1 cup warm milk (dairy or plant-based)

- Pinch cinnamon, 1 tsp honey

  Simmer 5 minutes. Drink before bed.

Quick Remedy	Safety Notes	Variations
Stir ashwagandha powder into warm milk.	Avoid during pregnancy. Use with caution if thyroid issues are present.	Add nutmeg for extra relaxation.

6. Peppermint Steam for Congestion

Why It Helps

Peppermint opens sinuses and eases colds or seasonal allergies.

How to Use

- 1 tsp dried peppermint
- 2 cups boiling water

  Pour into bowl, cover head with towel, inhale steam 5 minutes.

Quick Remedy	Safety Notes	Variations
Make peppermint tea and inhale steam while sipping.	Avoid steam burns. Not for children under 5.	Add thyme or eucalyptus leaves for stronger effect.

Pet-Friendly Healing

7. Chamomile Pet Calm Tea

Why It Helps

Chamomile calms anxiety in pets during thunderstorms or travel.

How to Use

- Brew weak chamomile tea (½ tsp dried chamomile in 1 cup hot water, steep 5 minutes, cool completely)
- Add 1–2 tbsp cooled tea to pet's water bowl

Quick Remedy	Safety Notes	Variations
Offer a few cooled drops by syringe for anxious pets.	Safe in small amounts for dogs. Avoid giving to cats in excess. Always consult a vet if unsure.	Lavender oil diffuser (out of reach) can calm pets too.

8. Calendula Wash for Pet Wounds

Why It Helps

Calendula is antimicrobial and promotes wound healing.

How to Use

- Brew 1 tbsp calendula flowers in 1 cup boiling water, steep 10 minutes, cool
- Use as wash for minor scrapes or irritations

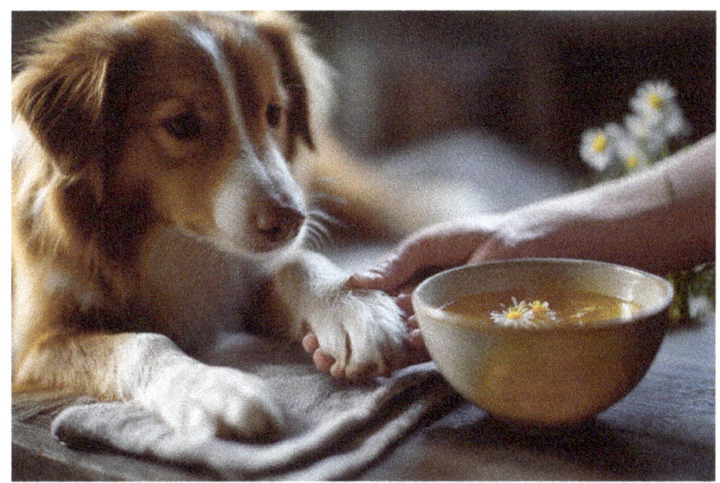

Quick Remedy	Safety Notes	Variations
Dilute calendula tincture with water (1:5 ratio) for a quick spray.	External use only. Avoid on deep wounds without vet care.	Combine with chamomile for inflamed skin.

Kitchen Cures

9. Garlic Honey for Colds

Why It Helps

Garlic contains allicin, an antimicrobial compound, while honey soothes throats.

How to Use

- Crush 6 garlic cloves
- Cover with raw honey in small jar
- Infuse 3 days before use
- Take 1 tsp daily or during colds

Quick Remedy	Safety Notes	Variations
Chew a raw garlic clove at first symptom.	Raw garlic may upset stomach.	Add ginger or cayenne for stronger remedy.

10. Ginger Tea for Nausea

Why It Helps

Ginger relieves nausea and supports digestion.

How to Use

- 1 inch fresh ginger root, sliced

- 1 cup hot water

  Simmer 10 minutes. Drink warm.

Quick Remedy	Safety Notes	Variations
Chew a thin slice of raw ginger.	Avoid large amounts if prone to reflux.	Add lemon and honey for extra soothing.

11. Cinnamon Honey Cough Syrup

Why It Helps

Cinnamon improves circulation, honey soothes the throat, and both have antimicrobial qualities.

How to Use

- Mix ½ cup raw honey with 1 tsp cinnamon powder

- Take 1 tsp as needed for cough or sore throat

Quick Remedy	Safety Notes	Variations
Stir cinnamon directly into warm honey.	Do not give honey to children under 1.	Add ginger powder for warming effect.

Making Family Healing a Ritual

The remedies in this chapter are more than instructions—they are invitations to ritual. Families thrive on routine, and weaving herbs into that rhythm helps children, partners, and even pets feel cared for in ways that are consistent and predictable. Ritual is what transforms a spoonful of syrup or a cup of tea from "medicine" into love.

Evening Family Tea Ritual

Why It Helps

Sharing tea together at the end of the day builds connection while gently supporting digestion, calm, and sleep. Herbs like chamomile, lemon balm, or oatstraw are mild enough for children yet soothing for adults.

How to Use

- Brew a large pot with 2 tbsp chamomile and 1 tbsp lemon balm in 4 cups hot water

- Steep 10 minutes, strain, and pour into mugs for each family member

- Sweeten lightly with honey for children over 1 year

Quick Remedy	Safety Notes	Variations
Use tea bags when evenings feel too rushed.	Avoid honey for children under 1 year; avoid chamomile if allergies are present.	Add rose petals for emotional balance or peppermint for after-dinner digestion.

 When my kids were young, bedtime was often chaotic. But when I began ending each evening with "family tea time," everything shifted. The children felt special having their own mugs, my husband enjoyed the moment of quiet, and I noticed fewer bedtime struggles. Years later, my daughter told me she now carries on this ritual with her own children.

Partner Connection: Herbal Massage Oil

Why It Helps

Touch is one of the most powerful medicines we can give one another. A simple herbal massage oil relieves sore muscles, reduces stress, and strengthens intimacy.

How to Use

Combine ½ cup olive oil with 2 tbsp dried lavender and 2 tbsp dried rosemary

* Warm gently in a double boiler for 1 hour, strain, and store in a glass jar
* Massage into shoulders, back, or feet after long days

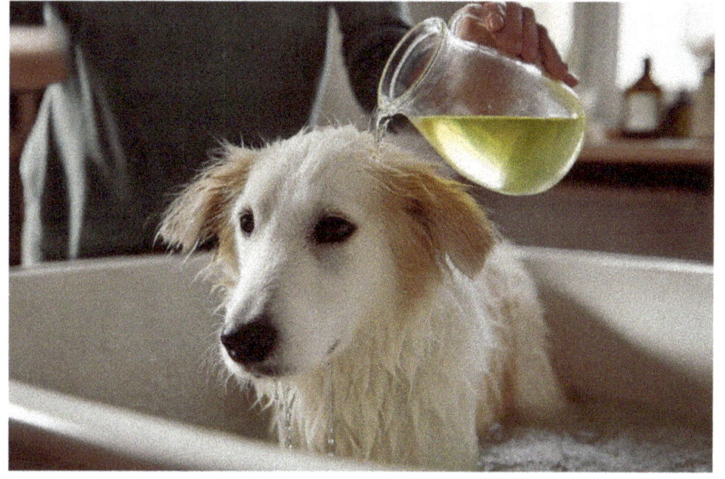

Quick Remedy	Safety Notes	Variations
Blend 5 drops lavender essential oil into 2 tbsp carrier oil if short on time.	Do not apply to broken skin. Test first for sensitivity.	Add arnica-infused oil for sore muscles or chamomile for deeper calm.

 My husband worked long hours at a physical job, and I remember his shoulders always felt like stone. Instead of just telling him to relax, I began warming a little lavender-rosemary oil in my palms and massaging his shoulders after dinner. It didn't just ease his tension—it became a ritual of connection. He said it made him feel cared for in a way words couldn't.

Pet Care Corner: Herbal Flea Rinse

Why It Helps

Herbal rinses can discourage fleas naturally, leaving coats shiny without harsh chemicals. Herbs like rosemary and lavender are safe in diluted form and create an inhospitable environment for pests.

How to Use

- Simmer 2 tbsp dried rosemary and 2 tbsp dried lavender in 2 cups water for 20 minutes
- Cool, strain, and pour over pet after a bath
- Towel dry, leaving rinse on the fur

Quick Remedy	Safety Notes	Variations
Dilute 2 drops lavender essential oil in 1 cup water, spray lightly on bedding.	Do not allow pets to ingest large amounts. Always monitor for sensitivity.	Add a pinch of sage or thyme for extra flea deterrent.

STORY FROM LYDIA: Our golden retriever, Willow, used to scratch constantly every summer. I hated using chemical flea treatments. When I tried an herbal rinse, not only did her itching reduce, but her fur smelled fresh and felt silky. Soon, bath time became part of her seasonal care, and the kids loved helping stir the herbs.

Kitchen Medicine Cabinet: Apple Cider Vinegar Tonic

Why It Helps

Apple cider vinegar (ACV) balances digestion, supports immunity, and can soothe sore throats when diluted. Families can use it daily in small doses for gentle support.

How to Use

- Mix 1 tbsp ACV with 1 cup warm water and 1 tsp honey
- Drink before meals or at first sign of sore throat

Quick Remedy	Safety Notes	Variations
Add a splash of ACV to salad dressings or soups.	Always dilute; undiluted vinegar can damage tooth enamel.	Infuse vinegar with garlic, onion, and ginger for a family-friendly "fire cider."

STORY FROM LYDIA: My mother swore by apple cider vinegar, and though I wrinkled my nose at the taste as a child, I now understand why. When my son went through a phase of constant sore throats, I began giving him diluted ACV with honey. Within days, his throat felt better, and he now keeps a bottle in his own kitchen as an adult.

Teaching Children the Healing Path

Children learn best by imitation. When they watch us tend herbs, brew teas, or rub balms, they understand healing as a normal part of life. I've found children are often eager helpers—they want to stir the infusion, count the drops, or sprinkle dried herbs into a jar. These small acts give them ownership and pride.

Practical Tips for Families:

* Let children choose their own tea mug and keep it as their "special healing cup."
* Invite them to pick herbs from a windowsill pot for dinner.
* Create a "family apothecary shelf" together, labeling jars with drawings or stickers.
* Encourage older children to keep a simple "healing journal" where they draw or write about remedies they tried.

These small acts turn herbs into part of family identity. One day, when your children are grown, they'll likely pass them on to their own families.

Reflection: Building Confidence Together

Many parents worry about doing it wrong. But remember: most of these remedies are food-based, safe, and simple. Trust grows with experience. Start with one herb and let your family grow familiar with it before adding more. Healing is not about perfection—it is about presence, love, and willingness to learn.

Bringing It Together

Earth medicine isn't just for you—it's for the ones you love. From child-safe chamomile teas to pet-friendly calendula washes, partner stress tonics to kitchen cures, each remedy in this chapter helps you extend healing into your family circle. These remedies are not complicated. They are simple, safe, and approachable, woven from ingredients you already recognize.

Start with one. Brew elderberry syrup this winter for your children. Rub arnica into your partner's sore shoulders. Add a splash of chamomile tea to your pet's water bowl. Each act is a reminder: you carry the power to nurture not just yourself but those around you.

When you turn the page, we'll explore how to deepen your relationship with earth medicine not just in moments of need but as a daily way of living, thriving, and belonging.

The Self-Heal Journey Is Yours

As we arrive at the end of this book, I want to remind you of something essential: this journey doesn't end here. In fact, this is only the beginning. The pages you've read, the remedies you've tried, the teas you've sipped—all of these are steppingstones. But the path of healing is yours, and it unfolds uniquely, in rhythm with your body, your family, your seasons, and your life.

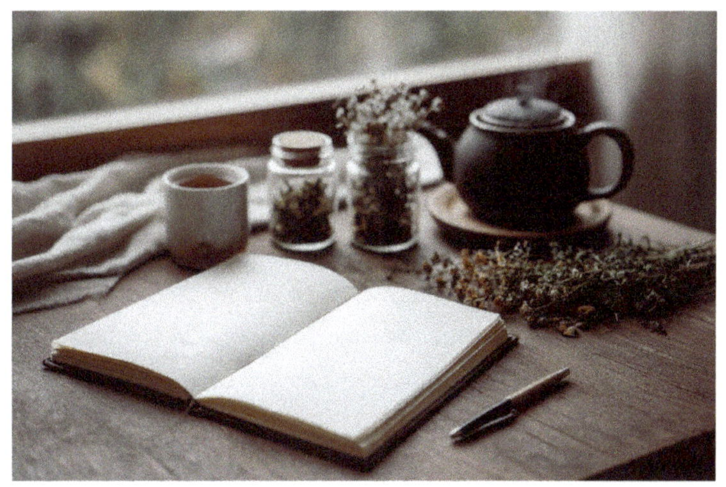

When people first pick up a book like this, they sometimes think they need to become a full-fledged "herb nerd"—someone with dozens of jars, hours of free time, and an encyclopedic memory of plant properties. I want you to hear me clearly: You don't need to be an expert to heal. You only need to begin.

I started, decades ago, with a single jar of chamomile and a single cup of tea. From there, I built confidence slowly. Healing isn't about knowing everything—it's about learning what works for *you*.

You Don't Need to Be a "Herb Nerd" to Heal

If you've ever scrolled through pictures of elaborate home apothecaries and thought, *"I could never do that,"* let this be your release. You don't need shelves of tinctures or rare ingredients to care for yourself. Healing begins in the kitchen, with a lemon and a cup of hot water. It begins in the garden, with a sprig of mint rubbed between your fingers. It begins on your windowsill, with a small pot of basil.

In fact, the simpler you keep it, the more likely you are to actually follow through. The truth is: healing sticks when it's easy, repeatable, and joyful.

You don't have to master every herb mentioned in this book. Instead, choose two or three that resonate with you right now. Maybe chamomile, nettle, and peppermint. Maybe lavender, garlic, and elderberry. Let those herbs become your allies. Build habits around them. As your confidence grows, you can add more. But even if you never move beyond those few herbs, you will still experience transformation.

Suggested Next Steps

Step 1: Build Confidence

Confidence grows not from knowing but from doing. Try one new ritual each week. Keep notes in a small journal—how you prepared it, how you felt afterward, what worked, what didn't. Over time, these notes become your personal handbook. You will begin to see patterns—what helps when you're stressed, what calms your digestion, what lifts your energy. This is how you begin to trust yourself as your own healer.

Step 2: Find Community

Healing becomes stronger in community. Look for local herbal workshops, farmers' markets, or online groups where people share their experiences. Ask questions, share your wins, and listen to others' stories. Even one friend who also enjoys tea rituals or simple remedies can make the path feel less lonely. In my own town, I've seen friendships bloom simply because two people began swapping jars of tea blends after yoga class.

Step 3: Keep Learning

If this book has sparked curiosity, follow it. There are endless ways to deepen your knowledge. You can take an online class, borrow books from the library, or attend a weekend workshop. Let your interest guide you. Some people fall in love with making salves, others with growing herbs, others with studying the history of plant medicine. Follow your joy.

The Real Work of Healing

When people ask me what the "secret" to natural healing is, I always smile. There is no secret. There's only the daily work of choosing yourself—again and again. I've had seasons where I was diligent with my oatstraw infusions, where my kitchen shelves overflowed with jars of golden calendula and deep green nettle. I've also had seasons where I let it all slip, too busy with work and family to remember even a simple tea.

But healing doesn't punish you for inconsistency. It waits. Like the mint plant in my garden that dies back in winter and returns in spring, herbs are patient. They are ready when you are ready. And your body is the same. No matter how long you've been disconnected, healing is always available when you return.

I want you to hold onto this truth: you cannot fail at healing. Every sip of tea, every drop of tincture, every slow breath is a victory.

Healing Across Life Stages

Herbal care looks different at different times of life. In my twenties, healing meant calming my anxious stomach before job interviews. In my thirties, it meant supporting my immune system through sleepless nights as a young mother. In my forties, it meant finding balance as hormones shifted and stress accumulated. Each decade brought new lessons, and herbs met me faithfully in each season.

Perhaps you are in your twenties, overwhelmed by career and new beginnings. Herbs like peppermint, lemon balm, and nettle will be your allies. Or maybe you are caring for children—then chamomile, elderberry, and oats will become your friends. If you are moving through menopause, herbs like sage, vitex, and ashwagandha will guide you through transition. And if you are tending aging parents, you may turn to hawthorn, garlic, and ginger to support their strength.

Your healing path will not look like mine, or your neighbor's, or your grandmother's. That is the beauty of self-healing—it adapts to you.

Overcoming Obstacles

Let's be honest: building healing habits isn't always easy. Life is demanding. You may forget to steep the tea. You may run out of herbs. You may feel silly carrying rosemary sprigs in your bag. That's okay.

Here are the most common obstacles I see and how to soften them:

* **"I don't have time."** Start with one-minute remedies. Lavender oil inhaled before bed, lemon squeezed into water in the morning. Healing doesn't require hours.

* **"I don't know enough."** You don't need to. Choose one herb and learn it well. Chamomile alone could support you for years. Knowledge builds naturally as you practice.

* **"I keep forgetting."** Use habit anchors. Pair your tea with brushing your teeth or lighting a candle. Place tinctures near your coffee pot or bed stand.

* **"I'm not consistent."** That's normal. Healing isn't about perfection. It's about returning, gently, each time you wander away.

The point is not to avoid obstacles—it's to learn to return anyway.

Final Ritual: The Deep Grounding Tea Ceremony

I invite you to make your tea ceremony not just a one-time act but a deeper initiation into your new way of living.

1. **Prepare Your Space.** Clear a small spot in your kitchen or living room. Light a candle, dim the lights, or place a small sprig of fresh herb nearby.
2. **Choose Your Herb.** Select one ally from this book that resonated most. Maybe nettle, lavender, chamomile, rosemary, or oatstraw.
3. **Brew with Intention.** Measure carefully. Pour the water slowly. Cover the cup, watching steam rise as though it carries your old patterns away.

4. **Sit in Stillness.** While the tea steeps, sit quietly. Place your hands on your heart or belly. Breathe deeply. Imagine the herb infusing not just your cup but your whole body with calm and vitality.

5. **Drink with Awareness.** Take the first sip slowly. Taste the layers. Imagine it traveling into your cells. With each sip, say silently: *"I am present. I am healing. I am whole."*

6. **Mark the Moment.** When the cup is empty, write one sentence in your journal: *"This is the day I chose my healing."* Date it. Let it anchor you whenever you forget.

This isn't just tea. It is a ceremony of becoming.

30-Day Healing Challenge

Here is a more detailed daily roadmap, filled with micro-actions that build confidence step by step. Each day is short and doable, but together they create lasting momentum.

Week 1: Awakening the Senses

- Day 1: Drink chamomile tea before bed.
- Day 2: Squeeze lemon into morning water.
- Day 3: Inhale rosemary or peppermint before work.
- Day 4: Journal one line about how you feel today.
- Day 5: Try 5 minutes of mindful breathing at lunch.
- Day 6: Add garlic to one meal with intention.
- Day 7: Reflect: What was your favorite moment of care this week?

Week 2: Nourishing the Body

- Day 8: Brew nettle infusion and sip throughout the day.
- Day 9: Replace afternoon coffee with peppermint or green tea.
- Day 10: Try one mineral-rich snack—pumpkin seeds or almonds.
- Day 11: Soak your feet in warm lavender water before bed.
- Day 12: Cook a simple soup with seasonal vegetables.
- Day 13: Write down one way your energy felt different this week.
- Day 14: Invite a family member to share tea with you.

Week 3: Rooting Rituals

- Day 15: Prepare elderberry syrup or buy pre-made and take your first spoonful.
- Day 16: Carry a lavender roller bottle in your bag.
- Day 17: Start a healing journal—dedicate a notebook.

* Day 18: Create a small apothecary shelf with two herbs.

* Day 19: Practice 4-7-8 breathing before bed.

* Day 20: Diffuse citrus oil in your workspace or home.

* Day 21: Reflect: How has your stress shifted since Day 1?

Week 4: Integration and Celebration

* Day 22: Brew tea for the whole family tonight.

* Day 23: Try one kitchen cure (like garlic honey or ginger tea).

* Day 24: Place a lavender sachet under your pillow.

* Day 25: Write a gratitude list of five things.

* Day 26: Step outside and put your bare feet on the ground.

* Day 27: Share a remedy or tip with a friend.

* Day 28: Journal: *"How do I want healing to feel in my life?"*

* Day 29: Repeat the grounding tea ceremony.

* Day 30: Celebrate. Reflect on the 30 days and note one ritual you want to continue.

By the end of this challenge, you will have tasted, smelled, touched, and lived with herbs every day for a month. This builds trust, memory, and most importantly—confidence.

Journaling Prompts for the Months Ahead

To carry your healing beyond this book, use these prompts each month:

* *This month, I noticed my body asking for…*

* *One ritual that felt supportive was…*

* *One thing that challenged me was…*

* *A lesson I want to carry forward is…*

* *Next month, I will…*

These questions keep you anchored in reflection, helping you celebrate wins and adjust with compassion.

A Seasonal Year of Self-Healing

One of the most beautiful ways to make your healing journey stick is to follow the seasons. Nature already gives us a rhythm, and when we align with it, healing feels less like a to-do list and more like a way of living. Here is a simple year-long guide you can adapt to your own life.

Spring: Awakening and Renewal

Spring is the season of fresh starts. As the earth greens again, our bodies also crave lightness and cleansing.

- **Herbs:** Dandelion, nettle, chickweed, cleavers
- **Foods:** Bitter greens, sprouts, radishes, asparagus
- **Rituals:** Brew a daily nettle infusion for minerals; try a simple dandelion salad once a week; step outside barefoot on soft ground as a daily reset
- **Reflection Prompt:** *What do I want to cleanse or release this season?*

Summer: Energy and Expansion

Summer is about vibrancy and outward energy. We sweat more, spend more time outside, and need hydration.

- **Herbs:** Mint, hibiscus, lemon balm, rose petals
- **Foods:** Watermelon, cucumbers, berries, fresh tomatoes
- **Rituals:** Sip hibiscus-rose iced tea in the afternoons; keep a lavender spritzer in your bag for hot days; journal outdoors in the evening light
- **Reflection Prompt:** *Where in my life do I want to shine more fully?*

Autumn: Grounding and Immunity

As the air cools, our bodies turn inward. This is the time to fortify the immune system and prepare for colder months.

- **Herbs:** Elderberry, astragalus, garlic, sage
- **Foods:** Squash, root vegetables, apples, oats
- **Rituals:** Make a batch of elderberry syrup for the family; simmer garlic and ginger in broth once a week; practice gratitude journaling as leaves fall.
- **Reflection Prompt:** *What do I want to preserve and protect as the year slows down?*

Winter: Rest and Restoration

Winter is the season of stillness. It is the time to rest deeply and nourish the nervous system.

- **Herbs:** Chamomile, ashwagandha, oatstraw, cinnamon
- **Foods:** Warming soups, porridges, spiced teas
- **Rituals:** Brew a nightly chamomile-oatstraw tea; rub your feet with warm sesame oil before bed; keep a candlelit tea ceremony once a week to mark the season.
- **Reflection Prompt:** *How can I allow myself to rest more fully this season?*

Monthly Micro-Rituals

To make it even easier, here's a suggestion of **one ritual per month** you can try:

- **January:** Start a nightly gratitude journal paired with chamomile tea.
- **February:** Make a heart-health tonic with hawthorn berries or garlic.
- **March:** Begin nettle infusions for mineral support.
- **April:** Add fresh dandelion greens to your meals
- **May:** Plant a pot of mint or basil on your windowsill.
- **June:** Keep a lavender spritzer nearby for calm in the heat.
- **July:** Brew hibiscus-rose iced tea for hydration.
- **August:** Try a simple mindfulness walk in nature once a week.
- **September:** Simmer elderberry syrup and stock your kitchen.
- **October:** Make a garlic-honey tonic to ward off colds.
- **November:** Practice a daily grounding breath before meals.
- **December:** Create a weekly candlelit tea ritual for rest.

By the end of the year, you'll have lived an entire cycle of herbal connection… one that grows deeper with each passing season.

Healing as Legacy: Passing down the stories and healing ways of my grandmother

When you choose to care for yourself with herbs, you are doing more than soothing today's stress or easing tonight's sleep. You are planting seeds of legacy. Every time you brew a cup of tea instead of reaching for quick fixes, you are showing your children, your friends, your community that healing can be simple, accessible, and joyful.

I still remember my grandmother's kitchen in Vermont. She didn't have a fancy apothecary, just jars of chamomile and peppermint she'd dried from the garden, and a crock of garlic honey on the counter. She would hand me a spoonful whenever my throat was sore. I didn't think much of it at the time. But decades later, when I make garlic honey for my own family, I realize I am carrying her wisdom forward. That is the power of herbal medicine: it ripples through generations quietly, lovingly.

Think of the little rituals you've built while reading this book. Maybe it's nettle tea in the morning, lavender oil at bedtime, or elderberry syrup each autumn. Imagine your children or grandchildren remembering those acts. Imagine your friends thinking of you when they brew their own tea because you once shared it with them. Healing habits don't just change your body—they shift the culture around you.

This is why consistency matters so much more than complexity. You don't have to master a hundred remedies or fill shelves with jars. Even one ritual practiced with love can leave a lasting imprint. When you choose to heal yourself gently, you are contributing to a quieter revolution: one where wellness is not bought in a bottle but grown in soil, shared in community, and sustained by care.

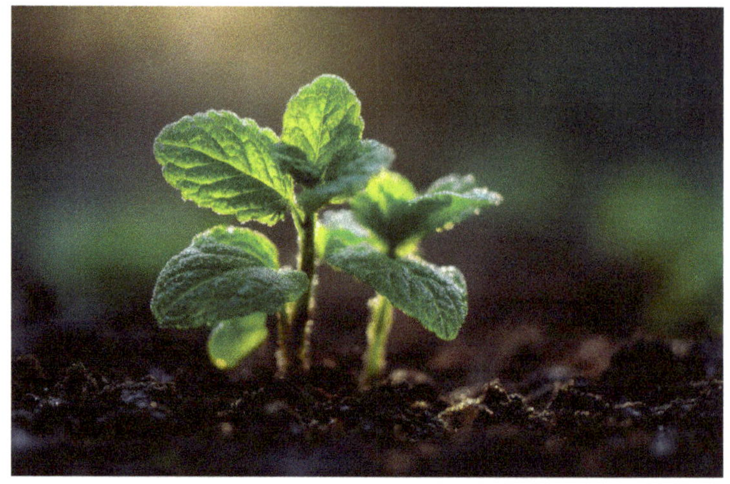

I want to encourage you to think of your healing journey not just as self-care but as **earth care and community care**. Each time you choose herbs, you are choosing to stay in relationship with the land. Each time you share a remedy, you are strengthening the bonds of your community. And each time you teach someone else—even by example—you are ensuring this knowledge is never lost.

So, ask yourself: *What do I want my healing legacy to be?* It might be as simple as teaching your child how to brew peppermint tea for an upset stomach. It might be tending a balcony garden and sharing mint cuttings with neighbors. It might be writing down your favorite remedies in a journal for someone to discover years from now. Whatever form it takes, trust that your healing journey extends far beyond you.

Closing Reflection

When I began writing this book, I thought of you—the reader who longs for simple remedies but feels intimidated, the parent who wants to care for their family naturally, the professional who worries they don't have time, the student who feels overwhelmed by too much information.

I want you to know that healing is yours. It belongs to you. It always has. Herbs are here to walk beside you, not to complicate your life but to simplify it. They meet you where you are: in your kitchen, your office, your city apartment, your garden.

Take what you've learned here and make it your own. Choose one herb, one ritual, one habit to carry forward. Let it grow roots in your daily life. Then, when you're ready, add another.

Your healing journey will not look like mine, and that's exactly right. This is your self-healing path. Walk it with curiosity, with gentleness, and with joy.

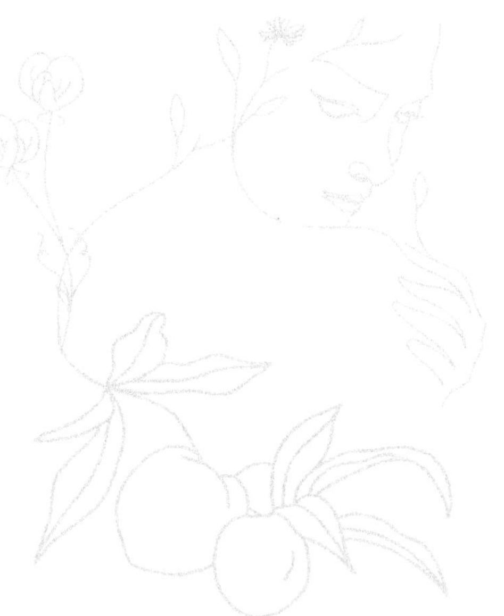

Further Resources & Community Guide

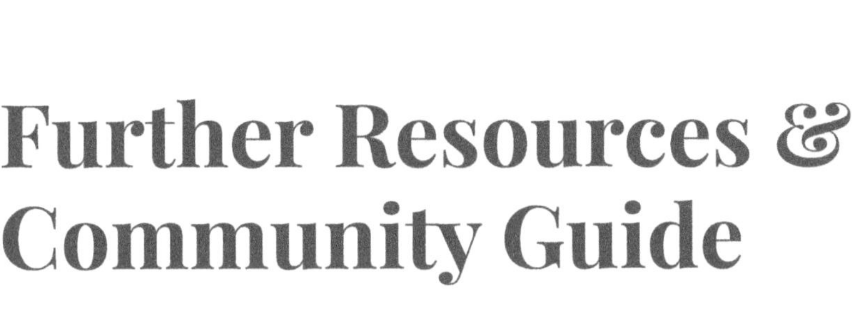

By now, you've learned dozens of remedies, practiced small rituals, and hopefully begun to trust yourself as a healer in your own life. But where do you go from here? Many readers tell me they want to keep learning, keep connecting, and keep building their confidence. This guide is here to offer you practical next steps.

Remember: You don't need to become an expert overnight. You are already a healer simply by caring for yourself and your loved ones. But if you feel drawn to deepen your knowledge, here are pathways to explore.

Books to Inspire & Teach

Books have been my greatest teachers. They allow us to sit at the feet of herbalists and healers who have walked this path for decades. Here are a few that I return to again and again:

- **Rosemary Gladstar's *Herbal Recipes for Vibrant Health*** — Rosemary has a gift for making herbs joyful, approachable, and deeply nourishing. Her recipes are simple enough for beginners yet timeless.

- **Sajah Popham's *Evolutionary Herbalism*** — For those who want to see herbs as bridges between body, spirit, and cosmos, Sajah offers profound insight into the patterns of plants.

- **Aviva Romm's *Botanical Medicine for Women's Health*** — A clear, evidence-informed guide for women's wellness across the lifespan.

- **Matthew Wood's *The Earthwise Herbal (Volumes I & II)*** — For readers who love story and folklore alongside clinical notes, these books are rich companions.

- **Anne McIntyre's *The Complete Herbal Tutor*** — A blend of modern science and traditional wisdom, great for building confidence step by step.

Keep in mind: you don't need to buy them all. Pick one that resonates, borrow it from your library, or even trade books with a friend.

Trusted Online Learning

Not everyone can travel to herbal schools, but online learning has made herbal wisdom accessible to all.

- **Herbal Academy** — Offers beginner-friendly courses with beautiful visuals, practical recipes, and a supportive student community.
- **Chestnut School of Herbal Medicine** — Based in the Appalachian mountains, their online programs include medicine-making and wild foraging.
- **Aviva Romm's Women's Health Programs** — Focused on women's wellness through evidence-based herbal and lifestyle care.
- **Evolutionary Herbalism** — Sajah and Whitney Popham's courses explore deeper plant-spirit connections and holistic energetics.

IF YOU choose to study further, take it at your own pace. Even a short introductory class can provide motivation and deepen your sense of belonging in the herbal world.

Finding Herbs & Supplies

You don't need rare or exotic plants to begin. Most remedies in this book can be made with common kitchen herbs and garden plants. But when you're ready to expand, here are some trusted sources:

- **Local Farmers' Markets & Co-ops** — Fresh herbs, local honey, and seasonal produce are often your best allies. Building relationships with farmers deepens your healing connection.
- **Bulk Herb Suppliers** — Mountain Rose Herbs, Frontier Co-op, and Starwest Botanicals all offer organic, ethically sourced herbs. Buying in bulk is cost-effective and lets you build your home apothecary.
- **Health Food Stores** — A simple way to find tinctures, teas, and essential oils. Look for products with clear sourcing and minimal additives.
- **Grow Your Own** — Even a windowsill garden with basil, mint, and thyme gives you fresh medicine at your fingertips.

Building Your Community

Herbalism thrives in community. Historically, women shared remedies over kitchen tables, grandmothers taught grandchildren to gather plants, and neighbors exchanged jars of salves. Today, we can recreate this spirit of connection.

Where to Look for Community:

- Local herbal workshops at libraries, yoga studios, or wellness centers
- Plant walks hosted by herbalists or community colleges
- Online forums and social media groups for herbal learning
- Community gardens where herbs are often planted and shared

How to Start Small:

- Invite a friend over for tea and swap stories about what's working for you.

- Organize a "remedy swap" where each person brings one jar of tea, syrup, or balm to trade.

- Create a seasonal ritual like "Spring Cleanse Tea" or "Autumn Elderberry Syrup Day" with friends or family.

Community keeps us accountable, inspired, and connected. Healing can feel isolating when done alone. But when you know others are also sipping tea or preparing remedies, you feel encouraged to keep going.

Your Herbal Learning Journal

One of the most powerful tools you can give yourself is a simple notebook. I call mine my **Herbal Learning Journal**. It is where I jot down:

- Recipes I've tried

- Notes on how remedies made me feel

- Seasonal reflections

- Stories from friends or community gatherings

- Sketches of plants I've met

Over time, this journal becomes your personal herbal book—unique to your body, your family, your landscape. No two journals will ever be the same. It is a way to trust your own wisdom, rather than always relying on someone else's words.

Passing It On

The greatest joy of herbalism is sharing it. When you brew a cup of chamomile tea for your child, you are teaching them that healing can be gentle. When you hand a jar of elderberry syrup to a neighbor, you remind them they are cared for. When you rub calendula balm on a scraped knee, you show your family that nature's medicine is always near.

This is how herbalism lives on—not in textbooks but in kitchens, gardens, and living rooms. By practicing and sharing, you become part of a lineage of healers stretching back through time.

Final Encouragement

You don't need to do this alone. You don't need to have it all figured out. Begin where you are, with what you have, and trust that herbs will meet you there.

Find a teacher. Find a friend. Join a group. Keep your journal. Share your remedies. And always, always return to the simple truth: **You are capable of healing, and you are never alone on this journey.**

References & Further Reading

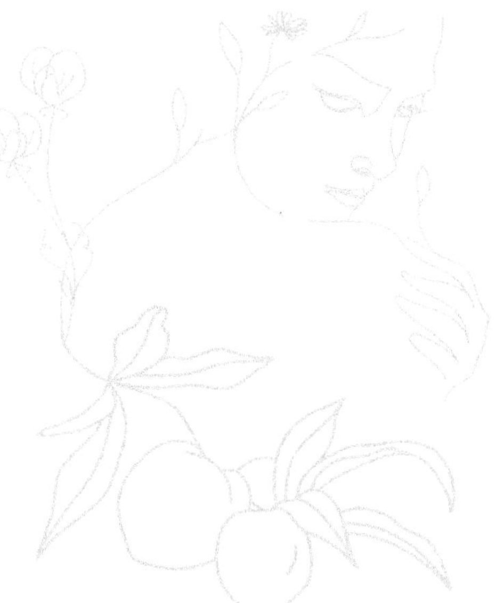

- Aviva Romm, *Botanical Medicine for Women's Health* (Churchill Livingstone, 2010)
- Rosemary Gladstar, *Herbal Recipes for Vibrant Health* (Storey Publishing, 2008)
- Rosemary Gladstar, *Medicinal Herbs: A Beginner's Guide* (Storey Publishing, 2012)
- Sajah Popham, *Evolutionary Herbalism: Science, Spirituality, and Medicine from the Heart of Nature* (North Atlantic Books, 2020)
- Matthew Wood, *The Earthwise Herbal: A Complete Guide to Old World Medicinal Plants* (North Atlantic Books, 2008)
- Matthew Wood, *The Earthwise Herbal: A Complete Guide to New World Medicinal Plants* (North Atlantic Books, 2009)
- Anne McIntyre, *The Complete Herbal Tutor* (Singing Dragon, 2013)
- Nicole Apelian, *The Lost Book of Herbal Remedies* (Claude Davis Publishing, 2019)
- Nicole Apelian, *Forgotten Home Apothecary* (Apelian, 2022)
- Phyllis A. Balch, *Prescription for Nutritional Healing, Sixth Edition* (Avery, 2010)